Colors in Homeopathy

NARAYANA VERLAG

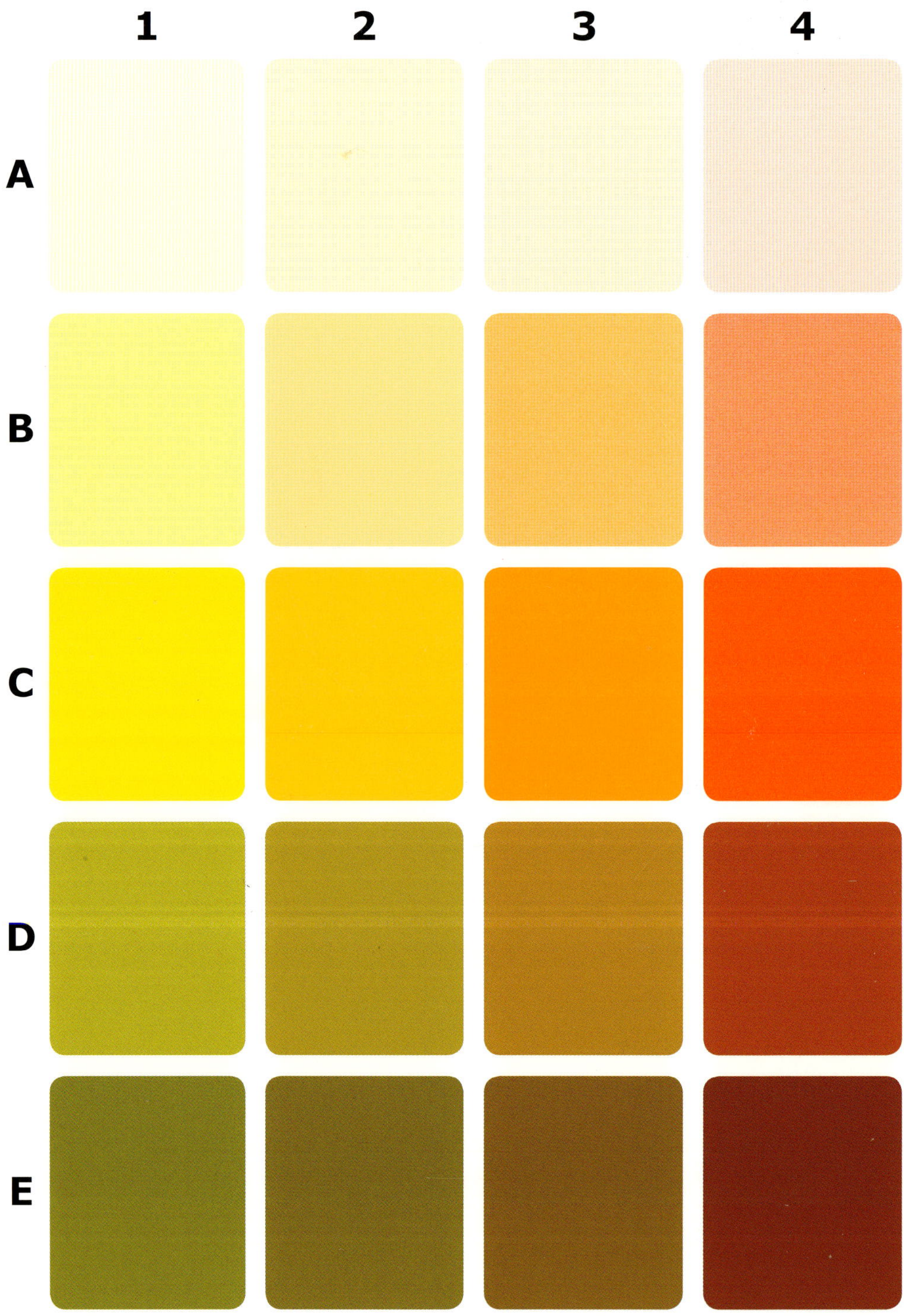
1
2
3
4
A
B
C
D
E

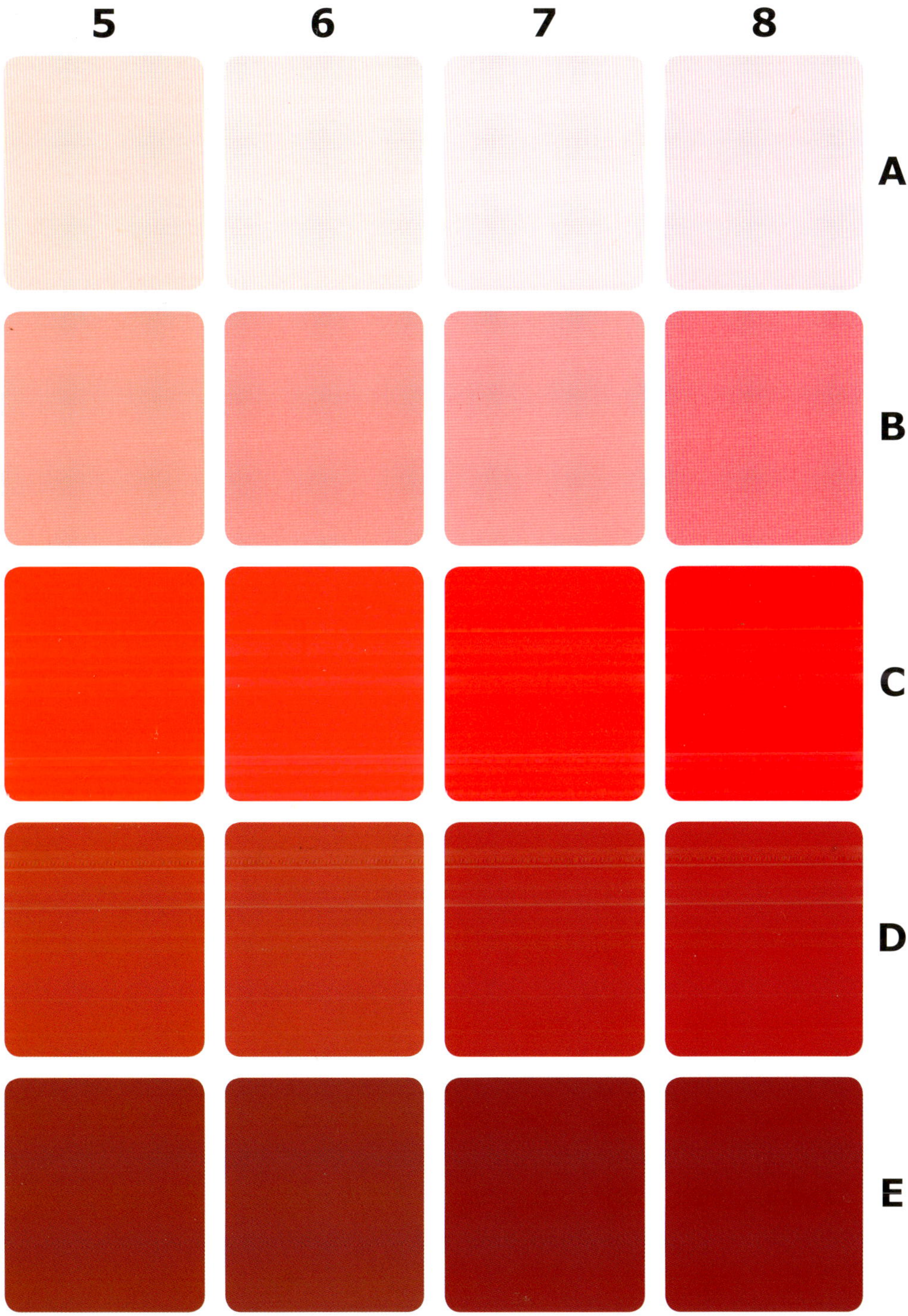
5
6
7
8
A
B
C
D
E

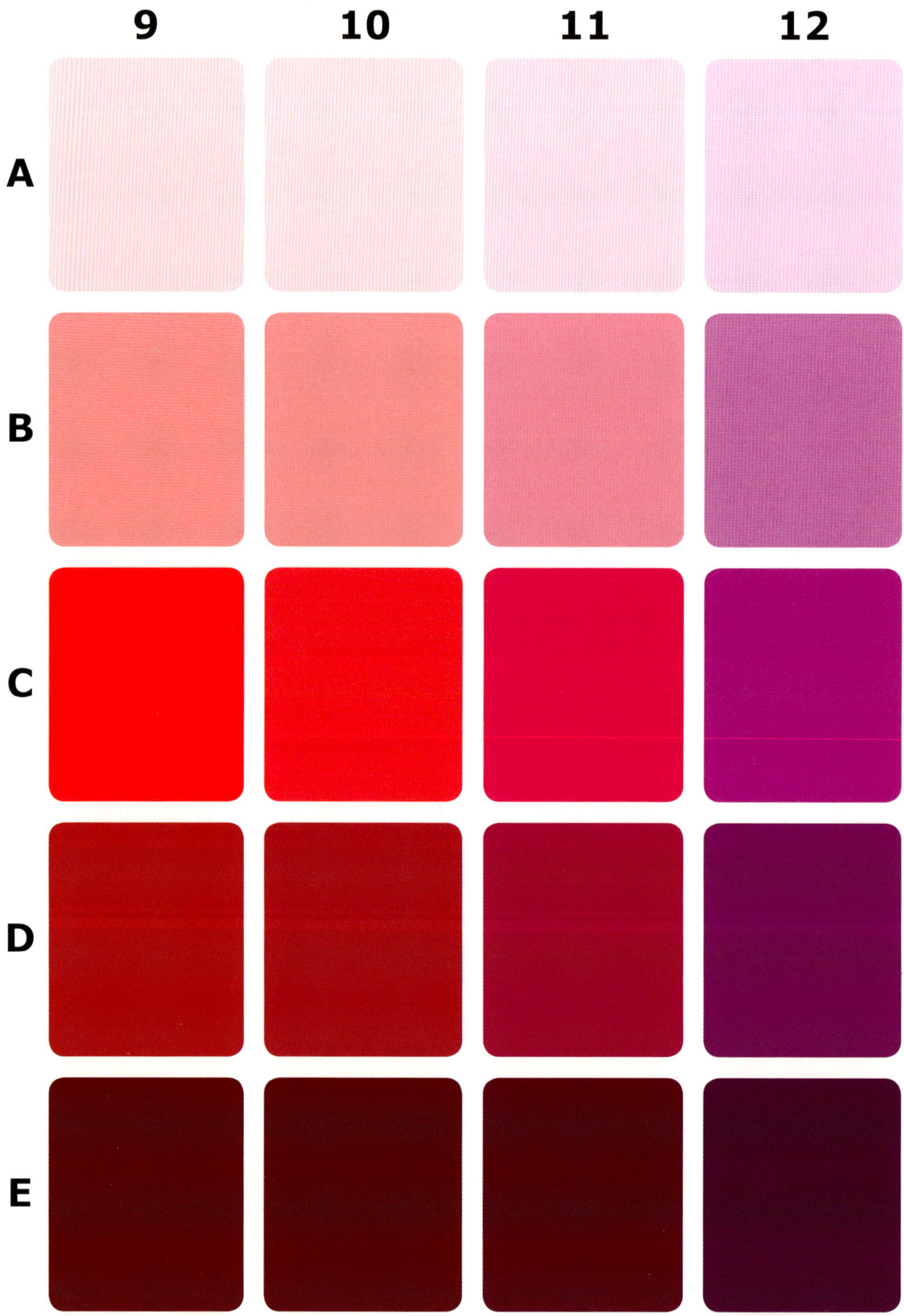
9
10
11
12
A
B
C
D
E

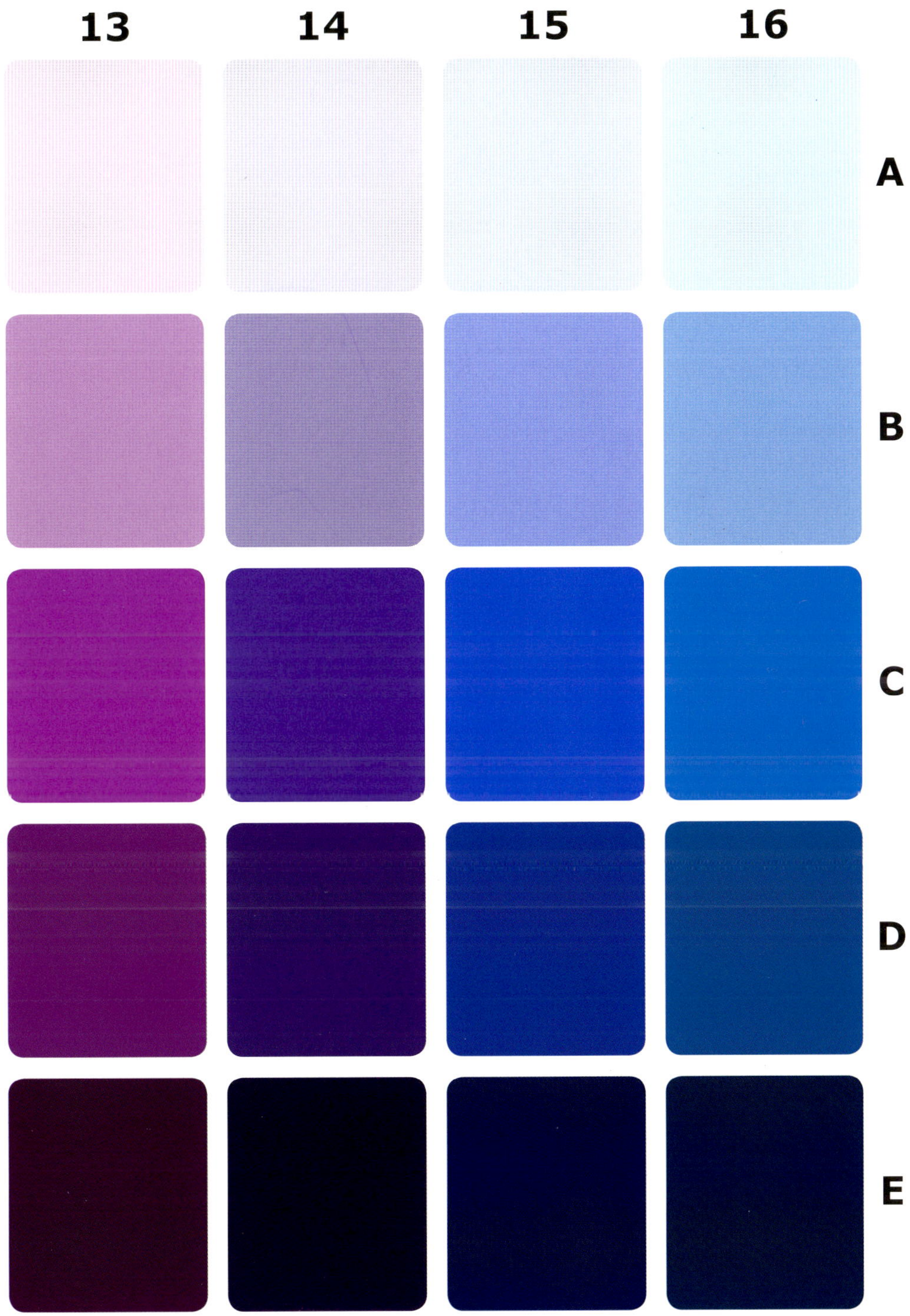
13
14
15
16
A
B
C
D
E

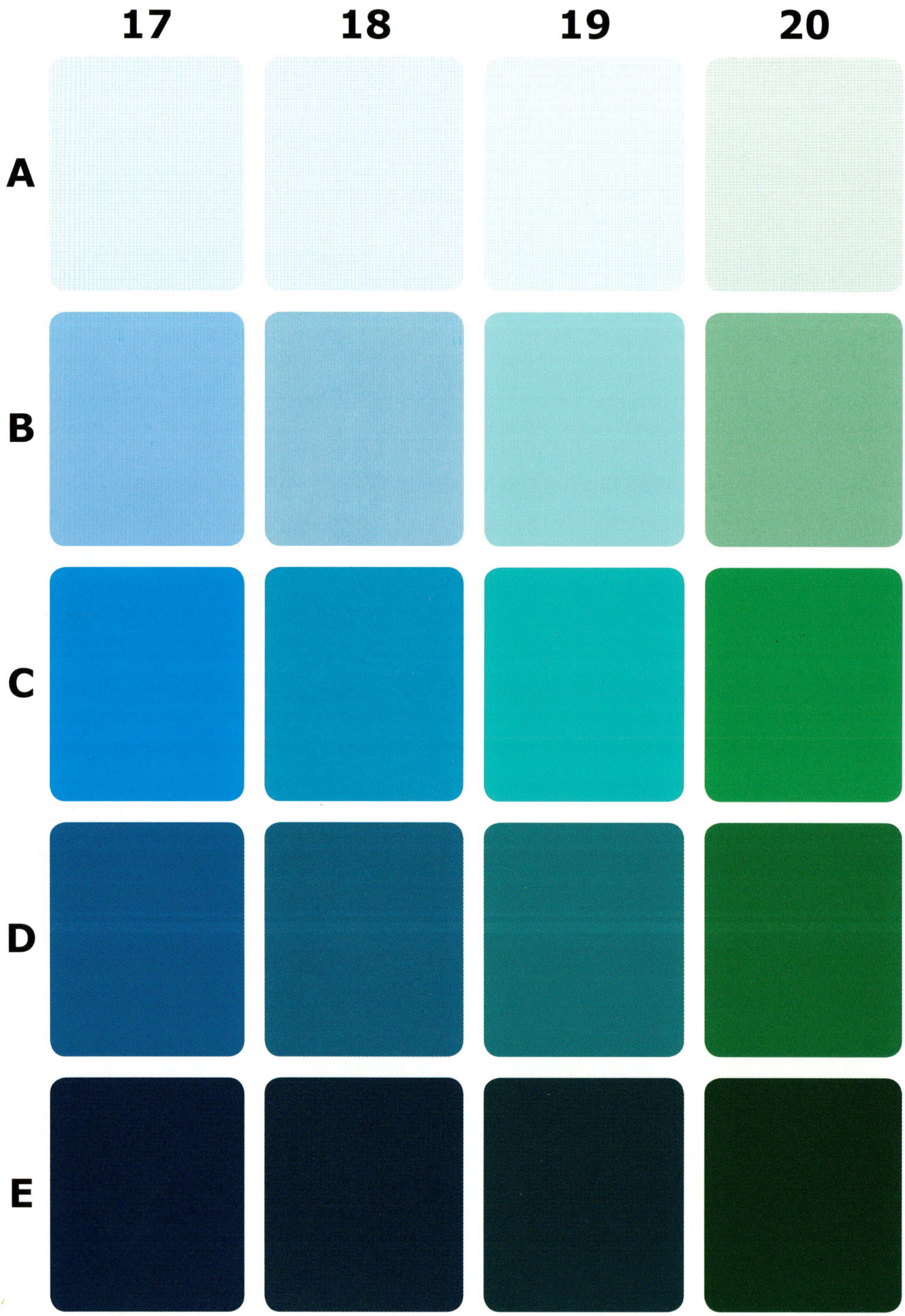
17
18
19
20
A
B
C
D
E

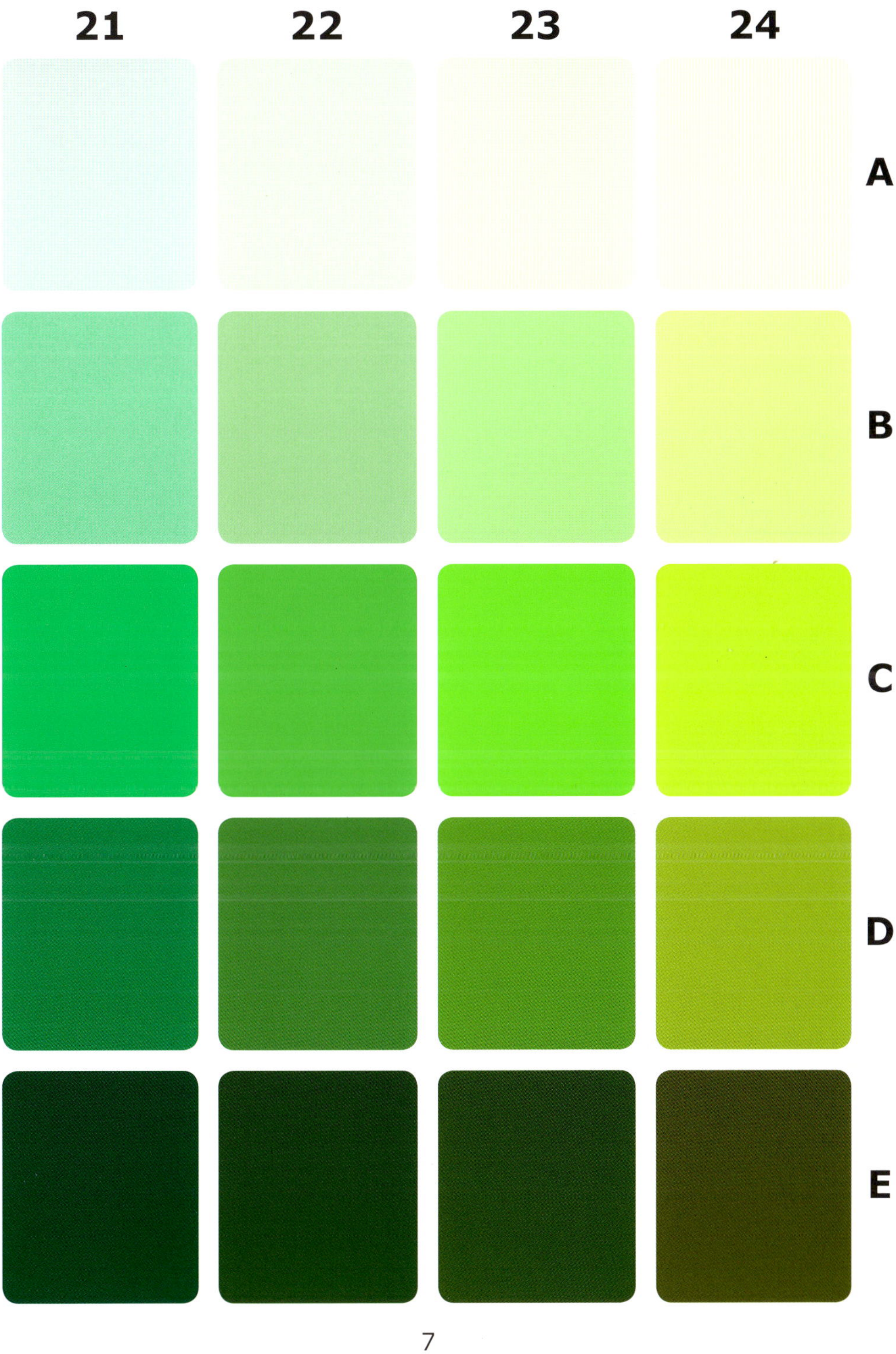
21
22
23
24
A
B
C
D
E

White **Black**

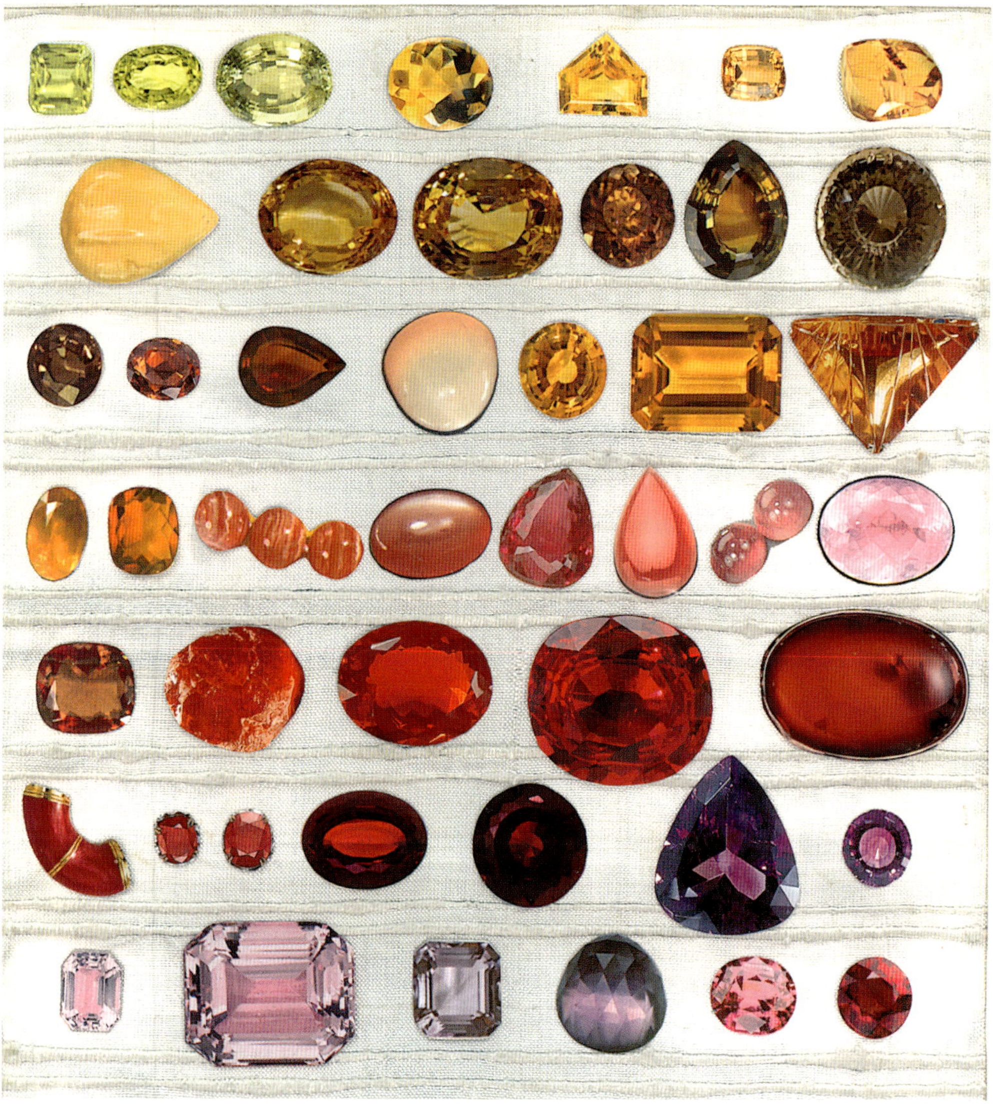

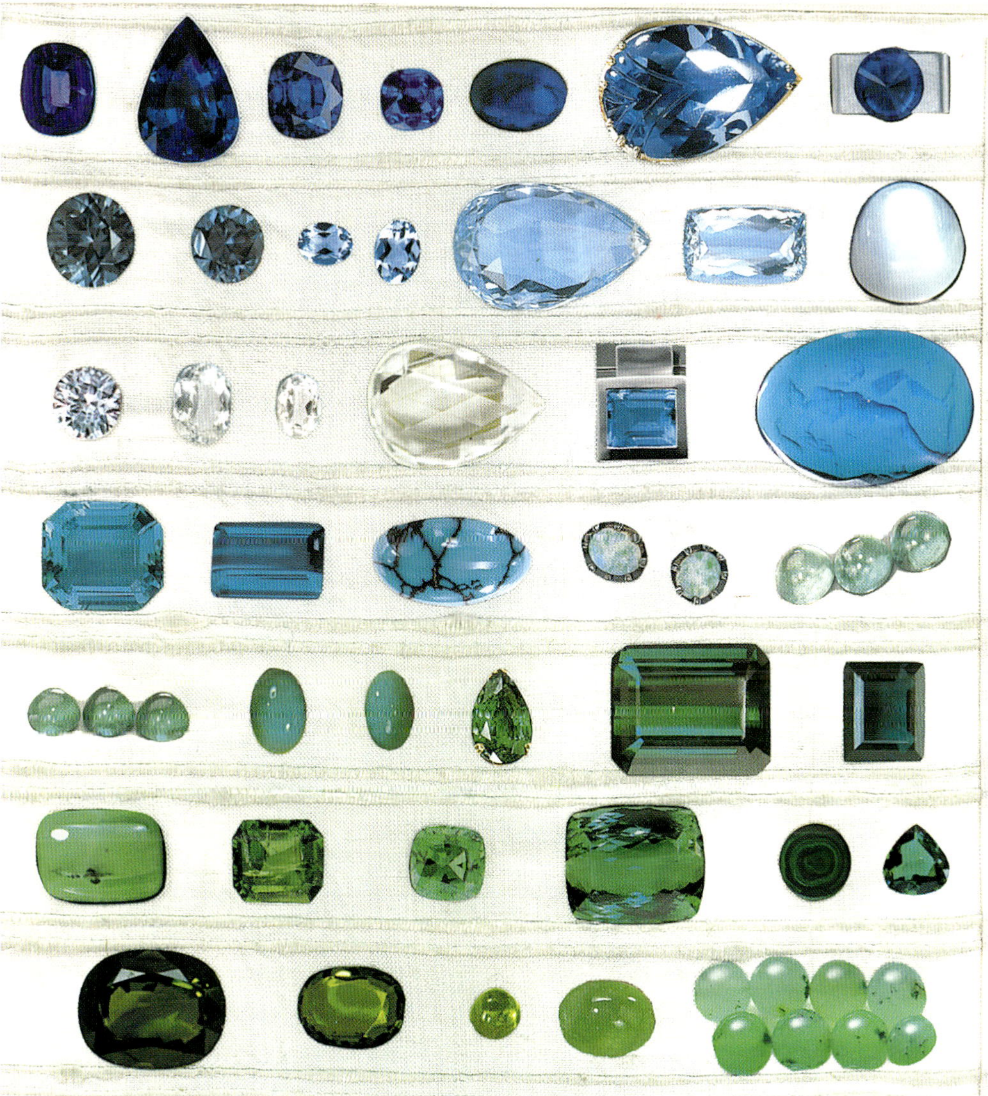

The list of remedies follows the abbreviations of Zandvoort's Complete Repertory. Only the remedies of the higher two degrees are given here: bold or 3rd degree for high confidence; plain type or 2nd degree for medium confidence, meaning at least two good cases with similar handwriting share the same color preference or – seldom – only one good case with high confidence of color preference. Many remedies follow Müller's grading but are not verified from us. As his grading has usually high accuracy we simply give it as it is. With many other remedies of 1st or lowest degree we have only 1-2 cases with uncertain color preference. We have omitted them here because the chance of error is still high. But if you want the latest suggestions for testing you can get the complete list under: www.homeo.de

Die Mittelliste folgt den Abkürzungen von Zandvoorts Complete Repertory. Wir geben hier nur die relativ sicher zugeteilten Mittel an: Dritter Grad oder Fettdruck bedeutet hohe Zuverlässigkeit, zweiter Grad oder Normaldruck steht für mittlere Zuverlässigkeit. Das heißt es gibt von dem Mittel mindestens 2 gute Fälle, die außer der gleichen Farbvorliebe auch eine ähnliche Handschrift teilen. Die Graduierung vieler Mittel folgt Müllers letzten Angaben und ist von uns noch nicht verifiziert worden. Da sie aber meist stimmen, haben wir sie mit wenigen Ausnahmen übernommen. Bei vielen anderen Mitteln, die im ersten (einfachsten) Grad stehen, haben wir nur 1-2 Fälle mit manchmal unsicherer Farbvorliebe. Wir haben sie deshalb hier nicht angegeben. Wer aber auch diese Suchfälle mit höherem Unsicherheitsfaktor nutzen will, kann die vollständige Liste einsehen unter: www.homeo.de

WHITE		**Alet**, **Alum**, Alum-met, **Apoc**, Apoc-a, **Arn**, Bell-p, **Croto-t**, **Dirc**, Eup-a, **Eup-per**, Eup-pur, **Solid**
GRAY		Rumx
BLACK		**Aeth**, **Arg-n**, **Bad**, Bamb-a, **Cic**, **Cic-m**, **Con**, **Graph**, **Grin**, Lac-eq, Luna, **Lycps**, **Oena**, Phel, Pitu-a
GOLD		**Anh**
YELLOW	1AB	Asar, Cich
	1C	Agar-ph, **Cann-i**, **Cann-s**, **Cur**, **Gels**, **Gnaph**, Gnaph-l, **Hyos**, Jatr, **Laur**, Lotus, Mand, **Nux-m**, Psil, **Symph**
	2A	**Hura**
	2B	**Agn**
	2C	**Agar**, Anac, **Bell**, Cham, **Chel**, **Clem**, **Ham**, **Ho**, Irid, **Op**, Penic, Petr, **Puls**, Sang, Tep, Upa
	3AB	**Verat**
	3C	**Aesc**, Botul, **Cer**, **Cham**, Esch, **Germ**, Gran, **Hell**, Ictod, **Ip**, **Lac-del**, Lachn, **Morph**, **Morph-m**, **Morph-s**, **Myris**, **Nux-v**, **Olnd**, Psor, **Senec**, Tanac, **Verat-v**, **Verb**
ORANGE	4-5C	**Brom**, Carb-ac, Cast-eq, **Chlol**, **Chlor**, **Chr**, **Euph**, Eupi, **Guai**, **Hydr-ac**, **Kreos**, **Lac-leo**, **Manc**, **Ph-ac**, **Sant**, **Sul-ac**, **Sumb**, Trib, Upa, Xan
BROWN	5E	**Am-c**, Am-caust, **Am-m**, Am-p, **Aral**, **Ars**, Ars-s-f, **Caust**, **Helo**, **Iber**, **Kalm**
RED	6C	**Calc-ar**, Chlam-tr, **Plat**, **Ptel**, **Saroth**, **Visc**
	6-11AB	Aloe, Anag, **Bov**, Chin-ar, Chin-m, Chin-s, Chin-sal, **Cycl**, **Epil**, **Ferr**, **Ferr-acet**, **Ferr-ar**, **Ferr-i**, Ferr-lact, **Ferr-m**, **Ferr-p**, Ferr-pic, **Ign**, **Sanic**
	7C	**Cact**, Calc-calc, **Dros**, Lac-v, **Staph**
	8C	**Apis**, **Bar-c**, **Bar-chl**, **Bar-cit**, **Bar-f**, **Bar-m**, **Bar-p**, Bar-s, **Calc**, **Calc-br**, **Calc-i**, Calc-lact, **Calc-m**, **Calc-s**, Calc-sil, Calo, **Carb-ac**, **Carb-an**, Chin, Cob, **Coloc**, **Gamb**, **Glon**, Guare, Hydrc, **Iod**, **Jab**, Lac-c, Mang-p, **Mur-ac**, Oxyg, Raph, Stroph, Stroph-s, **Sulf**, Vespa

RED	8-10D	**Calc-f**, **Calc-p**, Calc-sil, **Carbn-s**, **Carb-v**, Eupi, **Fl-ac**, Lac-c, **Lac-d**, **Thea**
	8-10E	**Abrot**, **Absin**, **Art-v**, Cina, **Hyper**, Lac-c, Lap-a, **Stram**, Syph
	9C	Adam, Chin-ar, **Merl**, Mim-p, **Sabad**, Vanad
	10C	Ferr-sil, Goss, **Hep**, Liatr, **Lup**, **Mill**, **Ran-b**, **Ran-fic**, **Ran-fl**, Ran-g, **Ran-s**, **Vinc**
VIOLET	11C-E	Ant-c, Ant-t, Borr-Nos, **Calen**, **Camph**, **Carbn-o**, **Dys-co**, Erb-n, **Hecla**, **Mang-acet**, Mang-c, **Mang-met**, Mang-p, **Morg**, Ox-ac, Pyrog, Sabad
	12-14AB	**Anan**, **Hist**
	12-14C	**Arist-cl**, Cocc, **Gent-l**, Gent-q, Heli, **Jug-c**, **Meny**, **Myric**, **Salv**, **Stann**, **Stront-br**, **Stront-c**, **Stront-i**, **Stront-n**, **Stront-p**
	12-14DE	Agra, **Aq-mar**, **Cadm-br**, **Cadm-m**, Cadm-p, **Cadm-s**, Cadm-sil, Murx, **Petr**, **Viol-o**
BLUE	15-16A	**Asar**, **Bapt**, **Grat**, **Kali-br**, **Kali-sil**, Mono-Nos, **Pityr-Nos**
	15-16B	**Colch**, **Cupr-ar**, **Kali-ar**, **Kali-p**, Led, **Plb-acet**, **Spig**, **Ust**
	15-16C	Abel, **Anthr**, Asperg-f, **Bac**, **Bamb-a**, Beryl, Beryl-c, Cob, Cocc, Coll, **Cop**, Corn, **Cupr-acet**, **Cupr-br**, **Cupr-c**, **Cupr-cy**, **Cupr-s**, Dicha, **Dig**, **Dios**, Dyspr-p, EBV-Nos, Erech, **Kali-bi**, **Kali-c**, **Kali-chl**, **Kali-cit**, **Kali-n**, **Kali-s**, **Lil-t**, **Lyss**, **Med**, Moly, **Onos**, Osm, **Pall**, **Phys**, **Plb**, **Plb-c**, **Plb-i**, **Plb-m**, **Rad-br**, **Rad-met**, **Rhod**, Sabal, **Salm-tp-Nos**, Samb, **Scan**, Ser-ang, **Tab**, Tax, **Teucr**, **Thal**, **Thal-s**, **Thuj**, Titan, Tril-p, Tung
	15-16D	**Ambr**, Beryl, Carc, **Cupr**, **Cupr-i**, **Cupr-m**, Dulc, Elae, **Kali-i**, Lycpr, **Pareir**, **Physal**, Physala-p, **Plb-p**, **Podo**, **Sec**, **Sol-c**, **Sol-n**, **Sol-t-ae**, **Tell**, **Tub**
	15-16E	**Caps**, **Cast**, **Eucal**, **Hydr**, **Osm**, Ox-ac, **Lyc**, **Medus**, **Paeon**, **Par**, Pic-ac, **Sep**, **Spong**, Techn

TURQUOISE	17AB	Nat-br, **Nat-c**, Zing
	17C	**All-c**, All-s, Ant-c, Ant-t, **Asc-t**, Chin-s, Lact, Lith-m, **Meli**, **Nat-m**, **Nat-s**, **Rhus-a**, Sinu-Nos, Squil
	17DE	Ant-o, Curc
	18AB	Anac, **Ant-s-aur**, **Nat-ar**, Nat-br, Nat-chl, Rhus-r, **Rhus-t**
	18C	Both-l, Dendro-p, **Elaps**, **Lac-f**, Lith-m, Naja, Nat-acet, **Nat-n**, **Nat-p**, **Rhus-c**, Rhus-r, **Rhus-v**
	18D	**Arum-m**, **Arum-t**, **Lith-citr**, Sieg, Zirk
	18E	**Cench**, **Lith-be**, **Lith-c**, SPS-Nos, **Vib**
	19AB	Bang-Nos, **Equis**, **Rauw**, Rob, **Sarr**, **Sin-n**, **Valer**
	19C	**Borx**, **Caul**, **Chin**, **Crot-h**, **Lach**, Naja, **Phyt**, Sym-r, Tus-p, Vip
	19DE	Borx, Lith-br, Lith-f, **Merc**, **Nat-be**, **Still**, Zirk
GREEN	20-22B	**Bufo**, **Coc-c**, **Daph**, **Ol-j**
	20-22C	**Acon**, Ail, **Allox**, Ang, Cinnb, **Cund**, Electr, **Helon**, **Hippoz**, **Ind**, **Mag-sil**, **Nitrog**, **Ol-an**, **Phos**, Sac-alb, Sil, **Tarax**
	20-22D	**Act-sp**, **Aster**, Aur, **Carc**, **Cimx**, M-aust, **Meph**, Merc-i-r, Moderhinke-Nos, Neuralgie-Nos, Ol-an, Ph-ac, **Rumx**, **Urt-u**
	20-22E	**Amyg-p**, **Asaf**, **Aur**, **Aur-br**, **Aur-m-k**, **Aur-m-n**, Aur-n, **Aur-s**, **Benz-ac**, Blatta, **Canth**, **Cimic**, Cinnb, Culx, **Cypr**, **Kohlhernie-Nos**, **Lob**, **Mag-c**, Mag-n, **Merc-cy**, Merc-i-r, **Plan**, Prun, **Psor**, **Rheum**, **Sil**
	23-24B	Coca, Com, **Croc**, **Euphr**
	23-24C	**Acet-ac**, Berb, **Bism**, **Bism-sal**, Brach, Cahin, **Coff**, **Mag-br**, **Mag-p**, Mand, **Mez**, **Mosch**, **Nit-ac**, **Nitro-o**, **Ruta**, Seneg, **Stry-ar**, Stry-i, **Stry-n**, **Stry-s**, **Zinc**, **Zinc-ar**, **Zinc-br**
OLIVE	23-24D	Card-m, **Iris**, **Mand-e-r**, **Rosm**, **Sabin**
	23-24E	**Elat**, **Mag-m**, **Mag-s**, **Tarent**
	1-2E	**Bry**, Bry-di, **Lat-m**, **Mygal**, **Syph**, **Ther**

A

Abel	15-16C
Abrot	**8-10E**
Absin	**8-10E**
Acet-ac	**23-24C**
Acon	**20-22C**
Act-sp	**20-22D**
Adam	9C
Aesc	**3C**
Aeth	**Black**
Agar	**2C**
Agar-ph	1C
Agn	**2B**
Agra	12-14DE
Ail	20-22C
Alet	**White**
All-c	**17C**
Allox	**20-22C**
All-s	17C
Aloe	6-11AB
Alum	**White**
Alum-met	White
Ambr	**15-16D**
Am-c	**5E**
Am-caust	5E
Am-m	**5E**
Am-p	5E
Amyg-p	**20-22E**
Anac	2C, 18AB
Anag	6-11AB
Anan	**12-14AB**
Ang	20-22C
Anh	**Gold**
Ant-c	11C-E, 17C
Anthr	**15-16C**
Ant-o	17DE
Ant-s-aur	**18AB**
Ant-t	11C-E, 17C
Apis	**8C**
Apoc	**White**
Apoc-a	White
Aq-mar	**12-14DE**
Aral	**5E**
Arg-n	**Black**
Arist-cl	**12-14C**
Arn	**White**
Ars	**5E**
Ars-s-f	5E
Art-v	**8-10E**
Arum-m	**18D**
Arum-t	**18D**
Asaf	**20-22E**
Asar	1AB, **15-16A**
Asc-t	**17C**
Asperg-f	15-16C
Aster	**20-22D**
Aur	20-22D, **20-22E**
Aur-br	**20-22E**
Aur-m-k	**20-22E**
Aur-m-n	**20-22E**
Aur-n	20-22E
Aur-s	**20-22E**

B

Bac	**15-16C**
Bad	**Black**
Bamb-a	Black, **15-16C**
Bang-Nos	19AB
Bapt	**15-16A**

Bar-c	**8C**
Bar-chl	**8C**
Bar-cit	**8C**
Bar-f	**8C**
Bar-m	**8C**
Bar-p	**8C**
Bar-s	8C
Bell	**2C**
Bell-p	White
Benz-ac	**20-22E**
Berb	23-24C
Beryl	15-16CD
Beryl-c	15-16C
Bism	**23-24C**
Bism-sal	**23-24C**
Blatta	20-22E
Borr-Nos	11C-E
Borx	**19C**, 19DE
Both-l	18C
Botul	3C
Bov	**6-11AB**
Brach	23-24C
Brom	**4-5C**
Bry	**1-2E**
Bry-di	1-2E
Bufo	**20-22B**

C

Cact	**7C**
Cadm-br	**12-14DE**
Cadm-m	**12-14DE**
Cadm-p	12-14DE
Cadm-s	**12-14DE**
Cadm-sil	12-14DE
Cahin	23-24C

Calc	**8C**
Calc-ar	**6C**
Calc-br	**8C**
Calc-calc	7C
Calc-f	**8-10D**
Calc-i	**8C**
Calc-lact	8C
Calc-m	**8C**
Calc-p	**8-10D**
Calc-s	**8C**
Calc-sil	8-10D
Calen	**11C-E**
Calo	8C
Camph	**11C-E**
Cann-i	**1C**
Cann-s	**1C**
Canth	**20-22E**
Caps	**15-16E**
Carb-ac	4-5C, **8C**
Carb-an	**8C**
Carbn-o	**11C-E**
Carbn-s	**8-10D**
Carb-v	**8-10D**
Carc	15-16D, **20-22D**
Card-m	23-24D
Cast	**15-16E**
Cast-eq	4-5C
Caul	**19C**
Caust	**5E**
Cench	**18E**
Cer	**3C**
Cham	2C, **3C**
Chel	**2C**
Chin	8C, **19C**

Chin-ar	6-11AB, 9C
Chin-m	6-11AB
Chin-s	6-11AB, 17C
Chin-sal	6-11AB
Chlam-tr	6C
Chlol	**4-5C**
Chlor	**4-5C**
Chr	**4-5C**
Cic	**Black**
Cich	1AB
Cic-m	**Black**
Cimic	**20-22E**
Cimx	**20-22D**
Cina	8-10E
Cinnb	20-22C,20-22E
Clem	**2C**
Cob	8C, 15-16C
Coca	23-24B
Cocc	12-14C,15-16C
Coc-c	**20-22B**
Coff	**23-24C**
Colch	**15-16B**
Coll	15-16C
Coloc	**8C**
Com	23-24B
Con	**Black**
Cop	**15-16C**
Corn	15-16C
Croc	**23-24B**
Crot-h	**19C**
Croto-t	**White**
Culx	20-22E
Cund	**20-22C**
Cupr	**15-16D**

Cupr-acet	**15-16C**
Cupr-ar	**15-16B**
Cupr-br	**15-16C**
Cupr-c	**15-16C**
Cupr-cy	**15-16C**
Cupr-i	**15-16D**
Cupr-m	**15-16D**
Cupr-s	**15-16C**
Cur	**1C**
Curc	17DE
Cycl	**6-11AB**
Cypr	**20-22E**

D

Daph	**20-22B**
Dendro-p	18C
Dicha	15-16C
Dig	**15-16C**
Dios	**15-16C**
Dirc	**White**
Dros	**7C**
Dulc	15-16D
Dys-co	**11C-E**
Dyspr-p	15-16C

E

EBV-Nos	15-16C
Elae	15-16D
Elaps	**18C**
Elat	**23-24E**
Electr	20-22C
Epil	**6-11AB**
Equis	**19AB**
Erb-n	11C-E
Erech	15-16C
Esch	3C

Eucal	**15-16E**
Eup-a	White
Eup-per	**White**
Eup-pur	White
Euph	**4-5C**
Euphr	**23-24B**
Eupi	4-5C, 8-10D

F

Ferr	**6-11AB**
Ferr-acet	**6-11AB**
Ferr-ar	**6-11AB**
Ferr-i	**6-11AB**
Ferr-lact	6-11AB
Ferr-m	**6-11AB**
Ferr-p	**6-11AB**
Ferr-pic	6-11AB
Ferr-sil	10C
Fl-ac	**8-10D**

G

Gamb	**8C**
Gels	**1C**
Gent-l	**12-14C**
Gent-q	12-14C
Germ	**3C**
Glon	**8C**
Gnaph	**1C**
Gnaph-l	1C
Goss	10C
Gran	3C
Graph	**Black**
Grat	**15-16A**
Grin	**Black**
Guai	**4-5C**
Guare	8C

H

Ham	**2C**
Hecla	**11C-E**
Heli	12-14C
Hell	**3C**
Helo	**5E**
Helon	**20-22C**
Hep	**10C**
Hippoz	**20-22C**
Hist	**12-14AB**
Ho	**2C**
Hura	**2A**
Hydr	**15-16E**
Hydr-ac	**4-5C**
Hydrc	8C
Hyos	**1C**
Hyper	**8-10E**

I

Iber	**5E**
Ictod	3C
Ign	**6-11AB**
Ind	**20-22C**
Iod	**8C**
Ip	**3C**
Irid	2C
Iris	**23-24D**

J

Jab	**8C**
Jatr	1C
Jug-c	**12-14C**

K

Kali-ar	**15-16B**
Kali-bi	**15-16C**

Kali-br	**15-16A**
Kali-c	**15-16C**
Kali-chl	**15-16C**
Kali-cit	**15-16C**
Kali-i	**15-16D**
Kali-n	**15-16C**
Kali-p	**15-16B**
Kali-s	**15-16C**
Kali-sil	**15-16A**
Kalm	**5E**
Kohlhernie-Nos	**20-22E**
Kreos	**4-5C**

L

Lac-c	8C, 8-10D
Lac-d	**8-10D**
Lac-del	**3C**
Lac-eq	Black
Lac-f	**18C**
Lach	**19C**
Lachn	3C
Lac-leo	**4-5C**
Lact	17C
Lac-v	7C
Lap-a	8-10E
Lat-m	**1-2E**
Laur	**1C**
Led	15-16BC
Liatr	10C
Lil-t	**15-16C**
Lith-be	**18E**
Lith-br	19DE
Lith-c	**18E**
Lith-citr	**18D**
Lith-f	19DE
Lith-m	17C, 18C
Lob	**20-22E**
Lotus	1C
Luna	Black
Lup	**10C**
Lyc	**15-16E**
Lycpr	15-16D
Lycps	**Black**
Lyss	**15-16C**

M

Mag-br	**23-24C**
Mag-c	**20-22E**
Mag-m	**23-24E**
Mag-n	20-22E
Mag-p	**23-24C**
Mag-s	**23-24E**
Mag-sil	**20-22C**
Manc	**4-5C**
Mand	1C, 23-24C
Mand-e-r	**23-24D**
Mang-acet	**11C-E**
Mang-c	11C-E
Mang-met	**11C-E**
Mang-p	8C, **11C-E**
Med	**15-16C**
Medus	**15-16E**
Meli	**17C**
Meny	**12-14C**
Meph	**20-22D**
Merc	**19DE**
Merc-cy	**20-22E**
Merc-i-r	20-22D, 20-22E
Merl	**9C**

Mez	**23-24C**
Mill	**10C**
Mim-p	9C
Moderhinke-Nos	20-22D
Moly	15-16C
Mono-Nos	15-16A
Morg	**11C-E**
Morph	**3C**
Morph-m	**3C**
Morph-s	**3C**
Mosch	**23-24C**
Mur-ac	**8C**
Murx	12-14DE
Mygal	**1-2E**
Myric	**12-14C**
Myris	**3C**

N

Naja	18C, 19C
Nat-acet	18C
Nat-ar	**18AB**
Nat-be	**19DE**
Nat-br	17AB, 18AB
Nat-c	**17AB**
Nat-chl	18AB
Nat-m	**17C**
Nat-n	**18C**
Nat-p	**18C**
Nat-s	**17C**
Neuralgie-Nos	20-22D
Nit-ac	**23-24C**
Nitrog	**20-22C**
Nitro-o	**23-24C**
Nux-m	**1C**
Nux-v	**3C**

O

Oena	**Black**
Ol-an	**20-22C**, 20-22D
Ol-j	**20-22B**
Olnd	**3C**
Onos	**15-16C**
Op	**2C**
Osm	15-16C, **15-16E**
Ox-ac	11C-E, 15-16E
Oxyg	8C

P

Paeon	**15-16E**
Pall	**15-16C**
Par	**15-16E**
Pareir	**15-16D**
Penic	2C
Petr	2C, **12-14DE**
Ph-ac	**4-5C**, 20-22D
Phel	Black
Phos	**20-22C**
Phys	**15-16C**
Physal	**15-16D**
Physala-p	15-16D
Phyt	**19C**
Pitu-a	Black
Pityr-Nos	**15-16A**
Plan	**20-22E**
Plat	**6C**
Plb	**15-16C**
Plb-acet	**15-16B**
Plb-c	**15-16C**
Plb-i	**15-16C**

Plb-m	**15-16C**
Plb-p	**15-16D**
Podo	**15-16D**
Prun	20-22E
Psil	1C
Psor	3C, **20-22E**
Ptel	**6C**
Puls	**2C**
Pyrog	11C-E

R

Rad-br	**15-16C**
Rad-met	**15-16C**
Ran-b	**10C**
Ran-fic	**10C**
Ran-fl	**10C**
Ran-g	10C
Ran-s	**10C**
Raph	8C
Rauw	**19AB**
Rheum	**20-22E**
Rhod	**15-16C**
Rhus-a	**17C**
Rhus-c	**18C**
Rhus-r	18C, 18AB
Rhus-t	**18AB**
Rhus-v	**18C**
Rob	19AB
Rosm	**23-24D**
Rumx	Gray
Ruta	**23-24C**

S

Sabad	**9C**, 11C-E
Sabal	15-16C
Sabin	**23-24D**
Sac-alb	20-22C
Salm-tp-Nos	**15-16C**
Salv	**12-14C**
Samb	15-16C
Sang	2C
Sanic	**6-11AB**
Sant	**4-5C**
Saroth	**6C**
Sarr	**19AB**
Scan	**15-16C**
Sec	**15-16D**
Senec	**3C**
Seneg	23-24C
Sep	**15-16E**
Ser-ang	15-16C
Sieg	18D
Sil	20-22C, **20-22E**
Sin-n	**19AB**
Sinu-Nos	17C
Sol-c	**15-16D**
Solid	**White**
Sol-n	**15-16D**
Sol-t-ae	**15-16D**
Spig	**15-16B**
Spong	**15-16E**
SPS-Nos	18E
Squil	17C
Stann	**12-14C**
Staph	**7C**
Still	**19DE**
Stram	**8-10E**
Stront-br	**12-14C**
Stront-c	**12-14C**

Stront-i	**12-14C**
Stront-n	**12-14C**
Stront-p	**12-14C**
Stroph	8C
Stroph-s	8C
Stry-ar	**23-24C**
Stry-i	23-24C
Stry-n	**23-24C**
Stry-s	**23-24C**
Sul-ac	**4-5C**
Sulf	**8C**
Sumb	**4-5C**
Symph	**1C**
Sym-r	19C
Syph	8-10E, **1-2E**

T

Tab	**15-16C**
Tanac	3C
Tarax	**20-22C**
Tarent	**23-24E**
Tax	15-16C
Techn	15-16E
Tell	**15-16D**
Tep	2C
Teucr	**15-16C**
Thal	**15-16C**
Thal-s	**15-16C**
Thea	**8-10D**
Ther	**1-2E**
Thuj	**15-16C**
Titan	Black, 15-16C
Trib	4-5C
Tril-p	15-16C
Tub	**15-16D**
Tung	15-16C
Tus-p	19C

U

Upa	2C, 4-5C
Urt-u	**20-22D**
Ust	**15-16B**

V

Valer	**19AB**
Vanad	9C
Verat	**3AB**
Verat-v	**3C**
Verb	**3C**
Vespa	8C
Vib	**18E**
Vinc	**10C**
Viol-o	**12-14DE**
Vip	19C
Visc	6C

X

Xan	4-5C

Z

Zinc	**23-24C**
Zinc-ar	**23-24C**
Zinc-br	**23-24C**
Zing	17AB
Zirk	18D, 19DE

Foreword by Jan Scholten

One of the biggest problems in homeopathy is the insecurity. Most prescriptions are not sufficiently grounded. Or better said the homeopathic diagnosis, which is the same as the remedy, is not sufficiently grounded. The result is that often the diagnosis turns out to be incorrect, the patient doesn't get better.

In order to increase the accuracy of the differential diagnosis we need confirmation. When we see a timid child with recurrent cold with mucus dripping from the nose we already know it may need Calcium carbonicum. To confirm the diagnosis of the remedy we need more symptoms. When we get them in the form of sweating on the scalp during sleep and desires for sweets and soft-boiled eggs our diagnosis is confirmed. The more confirmations we get, the more sure is the diagnosis and the result.

For confirmation it's good to have a broader range of symptoms. But especially peculiar symptoms, like the above desires. So how can we broaden our range of peculiar symptoms. One very good candidate is the color preference of a patient. Most patients can make a definite choice for one or more colors when offered a spectrum of colors. The color preference is a peculiar symptom expressing the inner state of the patient, which is the state of the remedy. And it's a specific symptom. The table of colors has 24 * 5 = 120 different colors, so it's very specific.

The German homeopath Hugbald Müller started with these concepts. This after he discovered that Conium not only has a desire for darkness, but also for the "color" black. His intuition led him to the idea that maybe every remedy will have its preference. He checked it and it turned out to be correct.

The writer of this book, Ulrich Welte, picked up the idea, together with his colleague Herbert Sigwart. Their Kandern clinic team confirmed the idea further. They gathered the color preferences of their patients over many years and found preferences for many remedies. An example is the little known remedy Cichorium intybus. With the color preference table it's possible to find the diagnosis of such a remedy. I think this is great.

The Kandern clinic team has greatly improved the color tables and enhanced the list of remedies. Müller used the "Taschenlexikon der Farben", but it has many disadvantages. The table designed by Ulrich Welte is the best usable I've seen till now. All colors are clear and accurately standardised, so it can be used in the future without ambiguity. All colors are represented. This means that almost every patient can find his color. Sometimes a patient will have a preference in between 2 colors. But also, as much important, is that there aren't too many colors. This makes it easier for the patient to have an overview. Irrelevant differences are left out. This is a great achievement that the writer could only accomplish with his experience of this symptom.

The color preference is a significant and effective symptom. It's effective in the sense that it can give the indication or confirmation of a diagnosis in many cases. What does that mean? It's again an indication of the primacy of the mind. Hahnemann called it Vital force, or dynamis, the invisible spiritual force behind all life. One can call it internal substance, spirit, inspiration, soul? The color preference as an expression of the inner state is closely connected with this vital force. It's an expression of the Mind, the Mind is ameliorated by the color, and that within seconds. The symptom of the color preference shows again the existence of a soul behind the body.

I hope we'll see more books of Ulrich Welte in the future, like the planned book on handwriting. This is again a new field for homeopathy and it will give us more possibilities for confirming our diagnosis.

Jan Scholten

The Color Preference as a Homeopathic Symptom

Introduction

Many people have a preference for certain colors. They may express it in clothing or articles of daily use. But there is a deeper side to it. If there is a color preference per se and unattached to purposes, we may regard it as a more general expression of the person's inner feeling. Thus it can become relevant for homeopathic use. In this sense the color preference can be seen as an individual basic state of the vital force, which expresses itself in a mental disposition.

The color preference has become a valuable symptom in our homeopathic work since 13 years, and we would not like to miss this additional information for a good prescription. The color preference is a symptom of great depth and relatively easy to get. We are convinced that the homeopathic profession irrespective of theoretical background can profit from it. It only requires an open mind with a truthful approach to the subject and enough patience to give it an earnest try. This book is the first genuine homeopathic color standard. It is meant as a daily desktop tool for finding and assessing the color preferences and then to use them as a homeopathic symptom. We did not spare any effort to give it the highest color printing quality and making it a fine and durable tool for easy use. The pages with all colors at a glance in the form of color circle, spectrum, and gem collection will make it easier to find the relevant color preference of the patient.

On reflection over this new publication we feel that the system is far from being complete, and every constructive input would be welcome. But at the same time we feel confident that our efforts will not go in vain and the wonderful science of homeopathy will profit by our endeavor. May the sapling grow and become a beautiful tree in the garden of homeopathy!

History

Dr. H.V. Müller from Cologne (1921 – 2001) discovered the homeopathic significance of the color preference around 1985. This hard-working and gentle soul initiated and perfected his new idea to a high degree along with his later discovery, the homeopathic significance of the handwriting. The idea of the color preference as a homeopathic symptom came to him initially from a Conium case. The patient was soothed by darkness (a known Conium symptom, but it is characteristic for more or less the whole botanical family, the apiaceae). The man also mentioned on his own accord that black was his favorite color. Then Müller began to look for it in other Conium cases. He saw that the color was confirmed, and thus the general idea of the color preference as a homeopathic symptom was born, ironically because of a color which is rather a negation of all colors. To work scientifically, he needed a common color standard by which one could define colors with sufficient diversity and accuracy. From the current available standards he chose the "Taschenlexikon der Farben" by Kornerup and Wanscher as the most appropriate, although it was not conceived for homeopathic use. With every patient he began to assess the color preference systematically, and he found that people cured by the same remedy often had exactly the same choice of color, even down to the same one color among the 1266 varieties of this book.

The idea appealed to us. But in his first publication he defined the color preferences of 26 remedies only, of which about half were so-called small remedies and seldom indicated. So we tried to find out the colors of more remedies on our own, but our first approach was a complete failure. The color preferences of our patients cured by the same remedy all differed, and we began to doubt the validity of the method in spite of some successful initial prescriptions. To get things clear we contacted Müller personally. He explained how to assess the colors and gave us a list of about 90 remedies the color preferences of which he had detected by then. That was at least a substantial number for individualized prescribing, and our successful prescriptions with the help of the color preference increased. Then we began to cooperate closely, and we contributed some new remedies also. We tried to improve the color tables, because the book had several shortcomings for homeopathic purposes. When he saw our new tools for an easier choice of color, he asked us in 1993 to publish a new homeopathic color standard, including new color tables plus color circle etc.

The main shortcomings of the old book were:

- The gamut of colors was overwhelming especially in the gray-tones and confused some people
- The red colors were not brilliant enough and kept many red-loving people from choosing them ("I cannot find my red among them")
- The turquoise part was insufficient, thus preventing for example the Natrium patients from finding their color
- The white pages in between the color pages were awkward for a comparative choice
- There was no section with all colors at a glance
- The book is out of print and will not be reprinted

The old book had split the color circle into 30 main colors and diversified these by 5 darker shades and 6 lighter tones each, a set-up according to the CieLab color space. Patients cured with the same remedy varied in their choice between 2-3 similar main colors especially in the violet, blue, and green sections. Thus the clinical significance of 30 main colors became doubtful and their number could be decreased. Müller gathered several similar colors into groups, and by years of experience the number of 30 main colors came down to 17 clinically relevant groups with their respective lighter and darker versions. If we had gone down to the rock bottom number of 17 major colors in the new book, the color circle would have looked awkward due to several gaps. We decided to go the middle way and omitted only the colors with the lowest clinical significance, but at the same time trying to keep a steady optical gradation from one color to the next. This gave enough smoothness to the color circle and an equal chance for every color. So the color circle came down to 24 main colors.

But the time from the idea unto the manifestation of the new book was long and beset with many difficulties. One of the main obstacles was the extremely high printing cost. The four color offset system is too limited for a reproduction of most of the desired colors. Only pure colors came into question. For optimum color effect we chose 21 Pantone colors and 3 HKS colors, but in the course of eight years three publishers refused because of the high costs. Then we decided to publish it on our own. So it took the book ten years to come into existence. And not least did it finally come to light due to the repeated requests of Jan Scholten. He had a beautiful hand in it and gave many valuable suggestions during the writing process also. Our deep felt thanks go with it.

How to get the favorite color of the patient?

The main thing is to get the full attention of the patient and his inner consent. If one succeeds in making him or her really interested to dive into the colors, with childlike simplicity if possible, we are likely to get the desired result. In a relaxed state, the patient should look at the color circle or spectrum, scan all the colors and then tell spontaneously in which area he feels best. Quite often intellectual preconceptions will try to intervene: why, how, for what shall I use the color? If a patient cannot let go of the idea to choose a color for clothes, then go with it, because it may also be the real color, although it deceives frequently. But if they are just uncertain what you mean, guide them gently away from any aspects of practical use, try to take them away from purposes and let them simply go to an area where they feel good, to a color that induces a pleasant feeling. Sometimes the exclusion of unpleasant colors can lead to the desired color.

If we see the patient for the first time, we wait until the regular anamnesis is over and the atmosphere is relaxed. This is a good moment to ask casually if they have a favorite color, a color one feels comfortable with, which pleases the eye. Then observe how he or she takes the question and how the answer comes. If it is natural and with thoughtful consideration, we can hand over the color book for an exact choice and note the code as first color. Another way is to give the color circle, spectrum or gem collection first and then only ask if they have any preference. Then only go into the detailed section. Please try different approaches and see which suits you best. Only mind that you get the interest and willing attention of the patient. Usually two colors will do.

Even a confident choice is only a good hint and no guarantee. Green-loving people are apt to change easily. Red and blue are the more determined and no-nonsense colors, the cornerstones of the visible spectrum between which the whole rainbow of colors spreads. In children the choice is relatively easy, if they can be made interested in the game. From around the age of 3 years, when they begin to prefer certain colors, we use a collection of balloons of different colors and make them choose one to keep. Or have a collection of little toys in different colors, color pencils etc. From around the age of four, they can also use the color book.

The choice of color should be repeated during the second consultation and possibly a third time after 3 – 6 months. We compare all colors chosen during different periods and see if one of them was re-chosen exactly in the same hue and lightness. This indicates a deeper color, which does not only represent a fleeting mood.

Experience has shown that in the majority of cases the limited selection of 5 shades of the 24 main colors facilitates the choice of the color preference, because many people get confused by too many color shades. But there are some who prefer a more detailed presentation. For this purpose the **Extended Color Table** was developed. This manual is a more sophisticated version of the present book and has the character of a precision tool. It is meant for the professional user desiring additional accuracy. It builds on the same 24 main colors but differentiates them in 19 different lighter and darker shades instead of only 5, thus presenting a total of 24 * 19 = 456 colors instead of 120. It allows a more subtle fine-tuning of the color preference.

From this extended version a separate poster, the **Extended Color Poster** (about 60 x 40 cm size) was created, which gives an overview of all the 456 colors. To see the continuity of the whole range of colors at a glance adds a new dimension to the perception of colors, which helps some people to find their color preference.

Difficulties

- *"I like all colors":* If a person likes all colors or wavers much, it can indicate that the real color preference is green (see Color Concepts). And if a decision seems too difficult we can ask for a favorite color of the past. Sometimes it gives a definite result. Or exclude some colors first and thus narrow the choice.
- *"I don't find my color here":* Then ask for the one, which comes closest to their real favorite. This can be a good indication, because they seem to know exactly what they want.
- *Too many questions:* If the patient asks too much about why and how and when, any choice will be doubtful. Such questions make things complicated and spoil every natural mood by far-fetched explanations and artificial constructs. We do not give much importance to the color then.

- *Trends of fashion:* The choice of color can be falsified by trends of fashion. Women sometimes choose their color of dress according to how they want to appear and not to how they feel. Sometimes the overdress is fashionable but the undercloth worn directly on the skin gives the true color preference. Or the choice of a jewel may give more clarity. They will often choose a gem according to their inner feeling. For this purpose we keep a collection of polished color stones, arranged in the succession of the color circle. Men sometimes give their color for cars, if they have a fancy for them.
- *Undecided:* If two or three colors have been chosen but the preference is uncertain, the chosen colors should be compared directly and noted in the given sequence. Frequently only a later repetition will clear it.
- *Painters etc:* Another difficulty frequently presents with people working with colors professionally or as a hobby. Sometimes a more frequent repetition of the color test gives one predominant color, but the value is doubtful.
- *Color blindness:* They also choose colors, but the result is doubtful. We lack experience with this subject.

Clinical reliability of the color preference as a homeopathic symptom

In July 2003, we made a retrospective study of 450 children up to 13 years treated successfully with a single remedy in our practice during the last 6 years. Of these, about 160 children were cured or improved by the usual homeopathic method and without the help of the color preference. The other 290 children had been old enough and willing to choose a color to their liking.

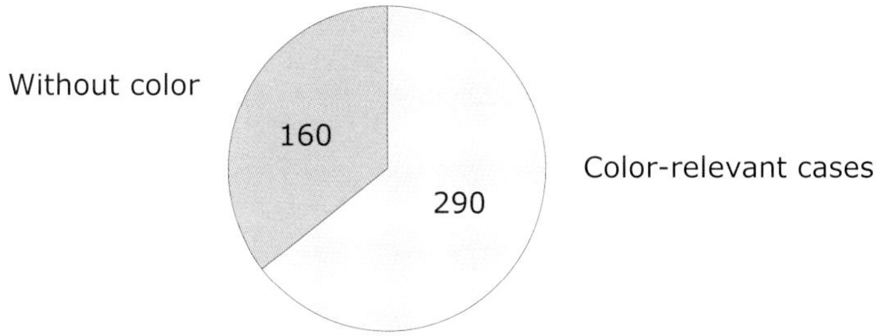

Total number of cases
n = 450

From this total number of 290 color-relevant cases, about 160 cases were solved with the help of the color preference. In other words, about 55% of these 290 children were cured or improved by a remedy found with the help of the color preference, i.e. one of two favorite colors matched with the color preference of the curative remedy. In about 30% of 290 color-relevant cases the given remedy was detected with the color preference as a leading symptom, meaning the color preference was the main symptom pointing to the remedy. And in about 25%, the color preference was a confirming symptom strengthening the choice made by the usual method (repertory symptoms etc). In these cases we could have arrived at the curative remedy without its help, although less certain. In the rest of the cases, about 45%, the color preference differed from the known color of the remedy (see diagram next page).

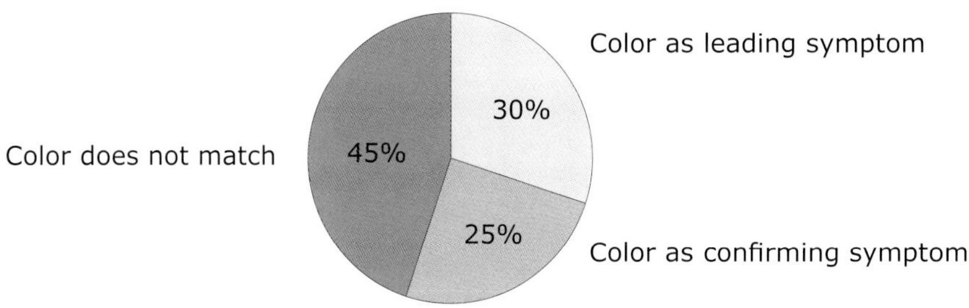

Color-relevant cases
n = 290

We do not think that these figures imply that the color preference could raise the success rate by 30%. We are rather of the opinion that one could have found other good remedies by other paths in many of these cases, although perhaps not always as good as the ones given. To prove or disprove these figures, an independent verification of experienced homeopaths is necessary. As we were using the already known color preferences, we were liable to take them for granted. It would be interesting indeed to get the color preferences of former good cases solved without this method, and we would welcome such cooperation.

Does the color preference change?

Yes, it can. We have seen this often in children. Their choice of color is usually easy and natural. You may repeat the color test frequently, but they remain with the same color preference even for some years, but then it may change suddenly. They enter another stage of development. We use this as an indication for another group of remedies.

Calendula: Let us take a case as an example. A girl aged three came with indurated, red and inflamed knots of the skin in both inguinal regions, bends of elbows and knees. The eruption was present since nine months. Six months before the knots appeared she had molluscae (a kind of warts) in the hollow of knees operated in full narcosis, because she resisted the operation so violently, that three men were not enough to hold her. She has an aversion to be touched by men, particularly by her father (who accidentally suffers from vitiligo all over the body). He wasn't supposed to even look at her in the morning. She was refined, charming, self-willed, and disliked any interference. She liked Barbie dolls and wanted to become a princess. She was much frightened by sudden piercing cries. She strongly disliked eggs. She chose the color 11 B, a rose pink. She got Calendula 1000 because of the asteraceae themes of her story (see Scholten's description of this family) and the color preference indicating particularly this variety of the asteraceae. No doubt, the prescription was not much more than a try, because the scanty proving symptoms of the remedy supplied no sufficient basis for a prescription. But it worked nicely. After 3 days the knots began to disappear, the inflamed parts healed. Then she got a high fever for one night only without feeling sick. Then she changed her attitude towards the father, and he was so surprised that he suspected her to be on drugs. She also started eating eggs and was less shocked by sudden noise.

She stayed exactly with the same color preference for seven months and then changed to 17 C, a cyan or bluish turquoise. This change of color came around the time when her father left the house and quit the family. Then she developed eczema of the chest. She got Nat-sil 1000 because of the father's withdrawal from home and leaving her alone[1], this being the suspected cause for her eczema. The new color

[1] See "Homeopathy and the Elements" by Jan Scholten, p. 233.

preference also pointed to the Natrium group. Within 2 weeks the eczema was gone, and she is fine since half a year now.

In some adults the color preference changes frequently, in others it stays the same for very long or even for life. Maybe they have found their permanent style, or their development might have got stuck due to power of settled habits and a loss of youthful vigor. The frequent repetition of the test itself seems to induce a superficial change of color in some people, and in these cases the result becomes doubtful. We feel that the main color with these people may be the first chosen during the first consultation, or it may be green (see Color Concepts). But those who like red or blue will remain with their choice for long, even if you ask them frequently.

Aversion to a particular color

Sometimes people have a definite aversion to a certain color. We think one should consider the same remedies as are given for this color as a preference, because it is just the other pole of the same axis. We have seen some cases supporting this idea, but we do not have much experience with it, because we did not ask systematically for color aversions. There are also cases of alternating aversion and preference to a particular color who were cured by a remedy given under this color as a preference. Maybe even the complementary color, i.e. the color placed in opposition in the color circle, can be used in the same way. But this third aspect is mere speculation. Please make your own experiments.

How to discover the color preference of a remedy?

During 15 years, an estimated number of 20 000 patients were asked for their color preferences. Of these, about 3000 patients contributed to the discovery of the color preferences of remedies, because they responded well to a certain remedy.

Cichorium: As an example, let us take a nice plant rather unknown in homeopathic circles and whose color preference was not known yet: Cichorium intybus, the wild chicory. Our aforementioned study of 450 children showed that we used 227 different curative single remedies. The most frequently used successful remedy was Belladonna in 10 cases, but Cichorium and Cina followed closely with 9 cases each. Nine cases cured by the same remedy are enough to define a color, and so we compared their data. As the color preference is a systematic integral part of our anamnesis, just like food modalities, the color codes from 6 of these 9 "Cichorium children" were noted in our case reports. 3 were too young to choose a color. The child who responded best to Cich had repeatedly chosen a very light and tender lemon yellow 1 A. The second best case had chosen exactly the same color, and one of five other fairly good cases chose a bit stronger lemon yellow 1 C. One fairly good case chose dark blue, and the least responding case chose dark violet, both approximately the complementary colors to light yellow (see Aversion to a color). Thus yellow emerged as the peak color of Cichorium, and to be more exact, it is a very light lemon yellow 1 A, or a bit stronger lemon yellow 1 C.

The leading symptom for the prescription of Cichorium, which was confirmed in six of our cases, was Scholten's information of the unwanted pregnancy, along with the characteristics of the asteraceae (compositae family). The mothers had initially thought of aborting the child. In four cases the children shrieked very loud and with a penetrating unpleasant voice. They were demanding, noisy and sometimes bossy, and they had a tendency for very high fevers. Seven of the 9 cases were good cases, not superficial ones. Thus we added Cich to our list in 2nd degree (a repertory evaluation, meaning it is confirmed at least by two good cases) under the color yellow 1 A. If more cases should confirm the color, it will get highest or 3rd degree.

The danger of overestimating the color preference

There was no chance for a bias towards the color preference in the aforementioned Cichorium cases, simply because the favorite color of the remedy was unknown. The remedy was prescribed in every case because of the usual symptoms, and the color preference played no part in the prescriptions. But in the Belladonna cases a certain bias towards the known color preference 2 C, a warm buttercup yellow, seems quite obvious. A homeopathic novice colleague chose the remedy frequently relying much on the easy color preference. With the result that 4 of the cases were of medium quality, just confirming a single set of symptoms or giving an isolated mental relief or curing a recurrent otitis without any deeper improvements. Prescribing on keynotes as a shortcut is one of the many homeopathic pathways, but its efficacy depends much on the quality of the used keynotes and if the essence of the case was properly understood. Relying on the color symptom indiscriminately will lead to failure. If we use the color only as one good symptom among others, adding to a full similarity of the remedy with the state of the patient, we will get better results.

Study of remedies by good cases

The retrospective analysis of a few real good cases cured by the same remedy can furnish an excellent opportunity for a deeper understanding of this remedy. Why should we rely exclusively on provings? Many new characteristics of remedies can be found by this clinical method also, provided we take only the real good cases. All color preferences were discovered retrospectively by meta-analysis of cured cases. The color preference is a clinical symptom. It does not come from provings, but it adds to the wealth of symptoms discovered by provings. H.V. Müller discovered the color preferences of hundreds of remedies by the clinical method. We confirmed many of them by fine cures. The complete list (including remedies only once verified and thus only mentioned for further tests) comprises about 700 remedies by now. We have experience with 550 of them, and the rest is given from Müller's experience exclusively.

Color preference and handwriting

The color preference is a subtle thing and can be quite evasive. Its assessment can be beset with several uncertainties (see Difficulties). So Müller began to search for another more solid symptom of individual relevance and hit upon the handwriting. From each patient he took a standardized sample on unlined A 4 paper and found similar writing structures in persons cured by the same remedy[2]. From around 1990, he began to cross the color preference with the handwriting as two new essential data to characterize a case from a personal level, along with the usual repertory rubrics from the homeopathic anamnesis. This combination gave more precision. In later years, Müller defined the color preference of a remedy only if he had at least two or three good cases sharing not only the same color

---

[2] It may be assumed that other general characteristics of remedies such as similar fingerprints, blood groups, DNA sequences, hand lines, iris patterns etc. could be found if we compare patients cured by the same remedy.

preference but also similar types of handwriting. But it narrows the definition of color preferences rather much.

Our correspondence used to be in the form of copied handwritings of cured patients on unlined sheets of A 4 paper. As a writing sample, the patients describe their main complaints or copy a standardized text. On the backside we give the medical diagnosis, color preferences and short indications for the remedy (repertory rubrics, materia medica symptoms, botanical concepts, series & stages, miasms etc). It will be out of place to write more on the subject here. We intend to write another book on the subject soon.

Can a remedy have several color preferences?

Müller was convinced that every remedy could have only one color preference. So most remedies in the list are mentioned only under one color. But there are reasons for a different view:

Bambusa arundinacea: Let us take an example. We have treated 11 patients successfully with Bambusa arundinacea, the bamboo. The prescriptions were based on an excellent proving with clinical verifications. From our cases we got the main color preference of bamboo, a lapis lazuli blue 15-16 C, and two types of well-corresponding handwritings. Six patients had chosen blue as their main color. Three others chose blue only as second color, one of them in a darker version 15 D. There was a second preference for black, although not as frequent as for blue. Three persons chose black as main color, and it was these who chose blue as second color. Other color preferences were randomly scattered, only green 20 C was chosen twice. Why then only give blue? Black should be mentioned as second color preference, because it stands out in these cases, although less pronounced.

The same two color preferences, blue and black, are the preferences of Titanium, but these patients have a different type of handwriting. In Manganum phosphoricum we have seen good cases with pure red or with a dark magenta as color preferences. Only more cases could tell how pronounced the given color preferences really are. Perhaps there are peaks of different colors with a stress on the main one in one remedy. Perhaps the combination of two colors is characteristic for some. Müller analyzed his cases in the same way as we describe it here, but he gave only the main color preference, perhaps to avoid further complications.

How do we use the color preference?

- *As a general symptom*: Normally we use the color preference like any other good general or mental symptom, with due care and with the readiness to dismiss it if other indications suggest a better remedy. The weight we give it depends on the concentration and certainty of the patient during the color choice.
- *In combination with the handwriting*: In choosing a remedy, one can compare the handwritings of all remedies given under the preferred color (of course you need a collection of handwritings for this method). If you find a similar writing type among one of these remedies, and the general characteristics of the case agree with the genius of the suggested remedy, you are quite sure to have a good prescription. If the general outlines of the remedy are confirmed by the personal characteristics of color preference and handwriting, we prescribe it with good confidence.
- *Differentiating similar remedies*: Say we have a case where it is difficult to see if Belladonna or Stramonium is more similar. If the color preference is red we would use Stram, if it is yellow we would give Bell.
- *Finding "small remedies"*: If you are in the habit of prescribing polychrests more frequently than lesser-known remedies, the color preference will frequently suggest the latter. Many colleagues told us that the color preference reminds them of small remedies and they would rarely think of them otherwise, because they are underrepresented in the repertories.
- *Computer repertorization*: One can introduce the colors in the computer repertorization, but if one uses the strategy of upgrading small remedies they will pop up as first even if there is no other reason for them but the color. So beware.
- *As a rescue symptom*: In case of difficult circumstances during the anamnesis like language problems, the color preference may sometimes come to the rescue. We had this experience in India and were surprised about the validity of the color. These cases were published in Homeopathic LINKS 1/01.

Color Concepts

This is a very promising field of homeopathic research. In this classification we see the key to a future natural system of themes and functions of the Vital Force. It will be based on the experience of the curative properties of remedies. Such a system would furnish a natural classification of remedies as well. We differentiate 4 main colors: yellow, red, blue, green; 3 intermediate colors: orange, violet, turquoise; 2 by-colors: brown, olive; and black and white, as well as its intermediate, gray. Thus we have a maximum of 12 groups, which can be defined as color concepts.

The theory of colors is an age-old subject, much debated and not generally agreed upon. Cultural differences may have an influence on the divergent views. Some scientific research has been done but with questionable results except for red and blue. The following versions are partly H.V. Müller's suggestions and partly our own observations. Especially the intermediate colors are still vague to us and so we have omitted them here. Please take the given concepts only as a working hypothesis and see for yourself.

Red Action Forward thinking, progressive Revolution Opportunism Passionate love Fire, heat	**Blue** Receptive Looking back, history Reaction Classic, reliable, conservative Boring Water, cooling
Green Change Variety Ambivalent Travel far Assimilation, growth	**Yellow** Imagination Inspired, high Clairvoyance Erratic, fickle Spaced out
Black No Independent I am the law Hard Dark power	**White** Pure like snow Disconnecting from passion Equalizing Hardened Radical

In conclusion

Finally it will not be out of place to reflect a little on the personal motives and circumstances of this work. As children of the sixties and influenced by the ideas, music and art of the hippie time, we met without knowing that fate would destine us to run a medical practice later on and to publish this book together. We were both keen on freedom through mental development and for religious experience in higher states of consciousness. Then we met a man who was an original thinker and writer and a great personality full of highest spiritual experience, which he knew to communicate in a joyful and most humble way. His name was Swami Narayanananda, and he emphasized the existence of a vital power called Kundalini Shakti, which is the dynamic aspect of quiescent consciousness. It is the source of mind, preserves its experiences in causal form and supplies them again as memory. The mind-functions depend on this vital force. It is the central bodily power and the very life of the body also. Without this vital force, the mind and body cannot exist[3]. When we realized some years later how closely Hahnemann's description of the vital force corresponded with the descriptions of this Saint it was but natural that homeopathy had a special attraction for us, and we started learning it in the mid seventies during the time of our medical education. In 1983 we started our joint clinic in the Black Forest in Kandern.

Hahnemann's idea of disease as a primal disturbance of the vital force expressing itself in physical and mental symptoms had caused much controversy, and we think it is partly due to a lack of abstraction from mechanical ideas. The vital force has no weight and no size and is beyond the conceptions of time and space, but, being the source of mind, it can be understood to a certain extent by a purified mind.

When the idea of the color preference as a homeopathic symptom was published, it appealed to us immediately as an easy-to-get symptom of great depth. Without much ado, it goes straight to the inner state of the person and gives suggestions of according remedies. It seems deeper or more general than a local symptom or a particular delusion (Sankaran's latest homeopathic researches in sensations and energy

[3] For further details, please refer to "The Primal Power in Man or the Kundalini Shakti" by Swami Narayanananda.

patterns point in the same direction). The color preference is a general disposition of the mind and roots in the individual vibration of the vital force. It differs according to the vibrations of the person's vital force and one may assume that it is connected to the individual aura. These vibrations "dye" the mind and one will take delight - or disgust, if the opposite is struck - in the correspondent colors. The color preference is of course not a disease but it may be connected to a disease like a particular soil favoring the growth of a particular weed.

Dear reader! Now we have come to the end of our story, and it would have served its purpose if you start using the book and gather your own experiences. May they be crowned with success for the benefit of your patients and for your own good in being able to help them!

Burgberg, August 2003

Ulrich Welte & Herbert Sigwart

Vorwort von Jan Scholten

Ein großes Problem der Homöopathie ist die Ungewissheit. Die meisten Verschreibungen sind zu ungenau begründet. Oder besser gesagt ist die homöopathische Diagnose, die ja dasselbe ist wie das Heilmittel, nicht genügend begründet. Im Nachhinein erweist sich die Diagnose oft als falsch, und dem Patienten geht es nicht besser.

Um die Genauigkeit der homöopathischen Differentialdiagnose zu verbessern, brauchen wir bestätigende Symptome. Wenn wir ein schüchternes Kind mit Infektanfälligkeit vor uns haben, dem der Schleim aus der Nase tropft, so weist uns das auf Calcium carbonicum hin. Wenn wir die Diagnose des Mittels sichern wollen, brauchen wir weitere Symptome. Falls wir hören, dass das Kind im Schlaf am Kopf schwitzt und gern Süßigkeiten und weichgekochte Eier isst, so ist unsere Diagnose gesichert. Je mehr bestätigende Symptome wir bekommen können, desto sicherer wird die Diagnose und das zu erwartende Resultat.

Zur Bestätigung ist es gut, wenn wir ein möglichst breites Spektrum von Symptomen haben. Besonders schätzen wir die charakteristischen Symptome wie zum Beispiel die genannten Nahrungsmodalitäten. Wie können wir also den Umfang unserer charakteristischen Symptome vergrößern. Ein ausgezeichneter Kandidat ist die Farbvorliebe des Patienten. Die meisten Patienten können sich für eine oder mehrere bestimmte Farben entscheiden, wenn man ihnen ein Farbspektrum vorlegt. Die Farbvorliebe ist ein charakteristisches Symptom der inneren Verfassung des Patienten und damit auch des gesuchten Heilmittels. Und sie ist ein spezifisches Symptom. Die Farbtabelle umfaßt 24 * 5 = 120 verschiedene Farben, also ist das Symptom sehr spezifisch.

Der deutsche homöopathische Arzt Hugbald V. Müller war der erste, der mit diesem Konzept zu arbeiten begann. Der Anlaß dazu war die Entdeckung, dass Conium nicht nur die Dunkelheit liebt, sondern auch die "Farbe" schwarz. Seine Intuition sagte ihm, dass möglicherweise jedes Mittel seine Farbvorliebe haben könnte. Er überprüfte es und sah, dass es stimmte.

Der Verfasser dieses Buches, Ulrich Welte, nahm den Gedanken auf, und zusammen mit seinem Praxiskollegen Herbert Sigwart bestätigten sie die Idee weiter. Sie sammelten die Farbvorlieben ihrer Patienten über viele Jahre hinweg und fanden die Farbvorlieben vieler Mittel. Ein Beispiel ist das wenig bekannte Mittel Cichorium intybus, die Wegwarte. Mit Hilfe der Farbvorliebe ist es möglich, auf die Diagnose dieses Mittels zu kommen. Ich finde das großartig.

Das Kanderner Praxisteam hat die Farbtabellen außerordentlich verbessert und die Liste der Mittel erweitert. Müller gebrauchte das "Taschenlexikon der Farben", doch es hat so manche Nachteile. Die Farbtabelle von Ulrich Welte ist die praktischste, die ich bisher gesehen habe. Alle Farben sind klar und genau standardisiert, so dass sie auch in Zukunft unzweideutig verwendbar sind. Alle Farben sind repräsentiert. Das heißt, dass fast jeder Patient seine Farbe finden kann. Manchmal wird die Farbvorliebe auch zwischen zwei Farben liegen. Ebenso wichtig ist, dass es nicht zu viele Farben gibt. Das erleichtert dem Patienten die Übersicht. Irrelevante Unterschiede wurden weggelassen. Die schwierige Entscheidung zwischen zu viel und zu wenig war nur möglich durch die langjährige Erfahrung des Autors mit diesem Symptom.

Die Farbvorliebe ist ein signifikantes und effektives Symptom. Effektiv in dem Sinne, dass sie in vielen Fällen die Bestätigung oder die Indikation zu einer Diagnose liefern kann. Was bedeutet das? Es ist ein weiterer Hinweis auf den Primat des Geistes. Hahnemann nannte es Lebenskraft oder Dynamis, die unsichtbare spirituelle Kraft, die hinter allem Leben steht. Man mag sie auch als innere Substanz, Geist, Inspiration oder Seele bezeichnen? Die Farbvorliebe als Ausdruck des inneren Zustands ist eng mit dieser Lebenskraft verbunden. Sie ist ein Ausdruck des Geistes, denn der Geist erlebt die Farbe als wohltuend, und dies innerhalb von Sekunden. Das Symptom der Farbvorliebe ist ein weiterer Hinweis auf die Existenz einer Seele hinter dem Körper.

Ich hoffe, dass wir bald weitere Bücher von Ulrich Welte sehen werden, wie das geplante Buch über die Handschrift. Das ist ein weiteres neues Feld für die Homöopathie und wird uns zusätzliche Möglichkeiten zur Sicherung der Diagnose an die Hand geben.

Jan Scholten

Die Farbvorliebe als homöopathisches Symptom

Einleitung

Wir haben meist eine gewisse Vorliebe für eine oder mehrere Farben. Das kann sich in der Kleidung oder in Gegenständen des täglichen Gebrauchs zeigen. Die Farbvorliebe kann aber auch der Ausdruck einer inneren Verfassung sein, die sich nicht auf Gegenstände beziehen muss. Spätestens dann ist sie homöopathisch verwertbar. In diesem Sinne kann man sie als Grundstimmung der Lebenskraft betrachten, die sich als geistige Neigung zu einer Farbe kundgibt.

Seit 13 Jahren hat uns die Farbvorliebe als homöopathisches Symptom so gute Dienste geleistet, dass wir sie als zusätzliche Information für eine gute Verschreibung nicht mehr missen möchten. Darum sind wir überzeugt, dass sie bei kunstgerechter Anwendung in jeder homöopathischen Praxis mit Gewinn eingesetzt werden kann, ganz gleich welcher Schule man folgen mag. Man braucht dazu nur einen offenen Geist, der nach wahren Fakten sucht, und etwas Geduld. Das vorliegende Buch ist der erste Farbstandard, der nach homöopathischen Gesichtspunkten konzipiert wurde. Er ist als tägliches Werkzeug gedacht, mit dem man die Farbvorlieben finden und genau genug bestimmen kann, um sie als homöopathisches Symptom in die Fallanalyse mit einzubinden. Wir haben in der Konzeption, im Druck und in der Herstellung keine Mühe und keine Kosten gescheut, um ein Werkzeug hoher Güte und einfachster Handhabung entstehen zu lassen. Der Farbkreis, die Übersichtstabelle aller Farben auf einen Blick und die Edelsteinsammlung erleichtern die gröbere Findung der Farbvorliebe, die dann in den Farbtabellen exakt definiert werden kann. Mit dem so gefundenen Farbcode kann man in den folgenden Tabellen die zugehörigen Mittel nachschlagen.

Trotz der relativ langen Reifezeit dieses Werks spüren wir nur allzu genau seine Unvollkommenheiten, und wir würden uns über jede konstruktive Mitarbeit freuen. Gleichzeitig sind wir überzeugt, dass die ganze Arbeit, die darin verborgen liegt, nicht vergeblich sein wird. Möge sie einen nützlichen Beitrag zum Wachstum der wunderbaren Wissenschaft der Homöopathie leisten!

Entdeckung und Entwicklung

Dr. H.V. Müller aus Köln (1921 – 2001) entdeckte die homöopathische Bedeutung der Farbvorliebe um 1985. Dieser liebenswürdige geniale homöopathische Arzt entwickelte die neue Idee zusammen mit seiner etwas späteren zweiten Entdeckung, der homöopathischen Auswertung der Handschrift, im Alleingang zu erstaunlicher Reife. Die erste Anregung kam von einem Coniumpatienten, der in der Dunkelheit Erleichterung fand. Dieses Coniumsymptom charakterisiert die meisten Vertreter der botanischen Familie der Apiaceae. In diesem Zusammenhang erwähnte der Mann von sich aus, dass schwarz seine Lieblingsfarbe sei. Darauf überprüfte Müller andere Coniumpatienten und fand diese Farbvorliebe bestätigt. So wurde die Idee ausgerechnet durch eine Farbe geboren, die eigentlich eine Negation aller Farben ist. Um wissenschaftlich arbeiten zu können, brauchte er einen allgemeingültigen Farbstandard, der eine genügend differenzierte und genaue Farbbestimmung ermöglichte. Er wählte das "Taschenlexikon der Farben" von Kornerup und Wanscher. Damit begann er systematisch bei jedem Patienten die Farbvorliebe zu definieren. Er fand heraus, dass viele Patienten, die mit derselben Arznei geheilt wurden, genau die gleiche Farbvorliebe hatten, und zwar zu einem Genauigkeitsgrad, der oft ein und dasselbe Farbfeld aus 1266 Farbnuancen traf.

Die Idee gefiel uns sofort, doch definierte er in seinem ersten Buch nur 26 Mittel mit ihrer zugehörigen Farbvorliebe. Die Hälfte davon waren kleine und eher selten indizierte Mittel. Also wollten wir selbst weitere Mittel farblich definieren. Der Versuch schlug gründlich fehl. Die Farbvorlieben unserer Patienten, die auf dasselbe Mittel gut angesprochen hatten, waren alle anders, und wir begannen am Wert der Methode trotz einiger anfänglicher erfolgreicher Verschreibungen zu zweifeln. Zur Klärung suchten wir Müller in seiner Praxis auf, und er zeigte uns, wie man die Farbvorliebe finden kann. Das ist nicht immer so einfach wie man meinen könnte. Ferner gab er uns eine Liste von ca. 90 Mitteln mit, die er inzwischen farblich definiert hatte. Diese Zahl war genügend groß, um differenzierter arbeiten zu können. Unsere Verschreibungsgenauigkeit mit Hilfe der Farbvorliebe wurde besser. Wir begannen, mit Müller enger zu kooperieren und konnten bald auch eigene Mitteldefinitionen beisteuern. Wir entwickelten neue Farbtabellen, weil das alte Buch, das nicht für homöopathische Zwecke konzipert war, einige Mängel aufwies. Als er unseren selbst entwickelten Farbkreis sah, bat er uns 1993, ein neues Farbenbuch speziell für homöopathische Zwecke herauszubringen.

Die Mängel des alten Farbstandards:

- Es gab zu viele Farben, und besonders die Graustufen waren für viele eher verwirrend als nützlich.
- Die Brillanz der Rottöne ließ zu wünschen übrig und hielt manche Rotliebhaber von ihrer Wahl ab.
- Der Türkisbereich war ungenügend differenziert, und die Natriumpatienten hatten Schwierigkeiten mit ihrer Farbe.
- Die weißen Zwischenseiten störten beim Farbvergleich.
- Es gab keine Übersichtstabellen aller Farben auf einen Blick.
- Das Buch ist außer Handel und wird nicht mehr aufgelegt.

Das frühere Buch unterteilte den Farbkreis im System des CieLab-Farbraumes in 30 Hauptfarben, die jeweils 5 dunklere und 6 hellere Töne aufwiesen. Nun zeigte sich, dass Patienten desselben Heilmittels in ihrer Farbvorliebe zwischen 2 bis 3 Hauptfarben variierten, besonders im Violett und im Blau sowie im Grünen. Damit war die klinische Signifikanz von 30 Hauptfarben in Frage gestellt. Müller begann mehrere Farben in Gruppen zusammenzufassen, und in jahrelangem Abgleich der klinischen Relevanz dieser Farbunterschiede schälten sich 17 Hauptfarben mit ihren jeweiligen helleren und dunkleren Tönungen heraus. Wenn man aber den Farbkreis auf diese 17 Farben reduziert, weist er mehrere optische Sprünge auf und wirkt unharmonisch. Daher gingen wir in der Auswahl der Hauptfarben den Weg der Mitte, ließen nur die Farben mit der geringsten klinischen Signifikanz weg und achteten auf eine gleichmäßige optische Abstufung von Farbe zu Farbe. So wirkt er mit 24 Hauptfarben ausgeglichen und gibt bei der Wahl allen Farben die gleiche Chance.

Vom Augenblick der Idee bis zum Druck war der Weg aber lang und voller Schwierigkeiten. Vor allem die hohen Druckkosten schreckten im Laufe von 8 Jahren insgesamt 3 Verleger ab. Das 4-Farben Offsetverfahren ist in seinem Farbraum zu begrenzt und kann die meisten gewünschten Nuancen nicht wiedergeben. So kamen nur Reinfarben in Frage, und in dieser Hinsicht gab es keine Kompromisse. Für einen optimalen Farbeffekt wählten wir 21 Pantonefarben und 3 HKS-Farben und entschlossen uns nach all den Ablehnungen zum Druck im Eigenverlag. Damit dauerte es 10 Jahre, bis die Idee verwirklicht wurde. Jan Scholten hatte entscheidend dazu beigetragen, denn er war es, der uns immer wieder darauf ansprach, das Buch herauszubringen. Auch im Entwicklungsprozess begleitete er das Werk und gab uns viele wertvolle Vorschläge. Unsere Freude über seine Mitarbeit begleitet das Buch.

Wie findet man die Farbvorliebe des Patienten?

Vor allem braucht man die volle Aufmerksamkeit des Patienten und seine innere Bereitschaft, sich auf die Farben einzulassen. Wenn es ihm gelingt, sich vorbehaltlos einfach in die Farben zu vertiefen, so werden wir das gewünschte Ergebnis bekommen. Der Patient oder die Patientin sollte die volle Aufmerksamkeit auf den Farbkreis oder das Farbspektrum richten, alle Farben überblicken und dann spontan den Bereich der angenehmsten Farbe angeben. Oft kommt gleich die Frage nach dem Wozu, Warum und Wie? Wenn unbedingt eine Farbe der Kleidung gewünscht wird, so mag sie manchmal die tatsächliche Farbvorliebe sein, doch besonders bei Frauen täuscht sie oft. Bei einer gewissen Unschlüssigkeit ist es besser, die Aufmerksamkeit sanft wegzuführen von gegenständlichem Nutzen. Am besten sucht man eine Farbe, bei der man sich einfach wohlfühlt und die das Auge erfreut. Manchmal kommt man auch durch Ausschluß von Farben zum Ziel, indem man den in Frage kommenden Rest immer mehr eingrenzt.

Wenn wir den Patienten noch nicht kennen, so warten wir, bis die Erstanamnese vorüber ist und sich eine entspannte Atmosphäre eingestellt hat. Dann ist der Zeitpunkt günstig für die beiläufig einfließende Frage, ob es eine Farbe gibt, die er mag und bei der er sich wohlfühlt. Man achte dabei, wie die Frage aufgenommen wird und wie die Antwort erfolgt. Kommt sie natürlich und nach einer gewissen Überlegung, so legen wir das Farbenbuch vor und lassen die genannte Farbe exakt bestimmen und notieren den Farbcode als Erstfarbe. Eine andere Methode ist es, zuerst den Farbkreis, das Spektrum oder die Edelsteinkollektion vorzulegen und dann zu fragen, ob eine bestimmte Farbe bevorzugt wird. Man stellt am besten eigene Versuche an und findet heraus, was einem am besten gelingt. Es kommt letztlich nur darauf an, das Interesse des Patienten zu wecken und seine Mitarbeit zu gewinnen. Zwei Farben genügen meistens.

Aber auch eine überzeugte Farbwahl ist nur ein guter Hinweis und keine Garantie. Grün als Farbe des Wandels neigt gern zu

Veränderungen. Rot und Blau sind eher feste und rationale Farben, sozusagen die stehenden Eckpfeiler, zwischen denen sich das gesamte Spektrum der Regenbogenfarben aufspannt. Bei Kindern ist die Farbwahl oft einfacher, wenn ihr Interesse an diesem Spiel erst einmal geweckt werden kann. Ab dem dritten Lebensjahr beginnen sie die Farben zu unterscheiden. Wir haben eine farbige Sammlung von Luftballons, unter denen sie einen wählen, den sie behalten und aufblasen dürfen. Oder man nimmt verschiedenfarbige Bauklötze, Farbstifte etc. Man kann ab dem 3. oder 4. Lebensjahr oft auch schon direkt das Farbenbuch nehmen.

Die Bestimmung der Farbvorlieben sollte bei der Zweitkonsultation und nach 3 bis 6 Monaten nochmals wiederholt werden. Wir vergleichen immer alle Farben und schauen, ob ein Farbton mehrfach exakt wiedergewählt wurde. Auch das kann ein Hinweis auf eine tiefere Farbvorliebe sein, selbst wenn sie nur als Zweit- oder Drittfarbe angegeben wurde.

Die Erfahrung zeigt, dass die Beschränkung auf je 5 Schattierungen bei den 24 Hauptfarben in den meisten Fällen die Auswahl der Farbvorliebe erleichtert. Zu viele Farbschattierungen wirken oft eher verwirrend. Doch gibt es auch einige Leute, welche eine detailliertere Präsentation bevorzugen. Aus diesem Grund wurde die **Erweiterte Farbtabelle** (“Extended Color Table**”**) entwickelt. Die erweiterte Farbtabelle ist eine separate Ergänzung des hier vorliegenden Buches und hat den Charakter eines Präzisionsinstruments, um erhöhte Genauigkeit bei der Farbauswahl zu erreichen. Sie gründet auf denselben 24 Hauptfarben, nur dass diese in 19 anstatt in nur 5 Schattierungen unterteilt sind. Dadurch ergibt sich die Gesamtzahl von 24 * 19 = 456 anstatt 120 Farben. Dies ermöglicht eine zusätzliche Verfeinerung der Farbauswahl.

Aus dieser erweiterten Variante des Farbenbuchs ging ein separates Poster hervor, die **Erweiterte Farbübersicht** (“Extended Color Poster” von ca. 60 x 40 cm Grösse), die einen Überblick über alle 456 Farben gibt. Das Wahrnehmen der fließenden Übergänge des gesamten Farbspektrums auf einen Blick eröffnet eine neue Dimension in der Bestimmung der Farbvorliebe.

Schwierigkeiten

- *"Ich liebe alle Farben":* Wenn jemand alle Farben mag oder häufig wechselt, kann es bedeuten, dass eigentlich grün bevorzugt wird (siehe Farbkonzepte). Wenn aber die Entscheidung trotzdem schwer fällt, kann man nach einer Farbvorliebe der Vergangenheit fragen. Oder man grenzt zuerst alle nicht in Frage kommenden Farben aus.
- *"Ich finde meine Farbe hier nicht genau":* Man frage dann nach einer Farbe, die der gewünschten noch am nächsten kommt. Das kann eine gute Indikation sein, denn diese Leute scheinen genau zu wissen, was sie wollen.
- *Zu viele Fragen:* Wenn ständig nach dem Warum, Wozu und Wann gefragt wird, so ist die Farbvorliebe meist dubios. Solche Fragen komplizieren alles und verderben jede natürliche Regung mit ihrem künstlichen Erklärungszwang.
- *Modetrends:* Die Farbvorliebe kann durch Modetrends überlagert sein. Frauen wählen ihre Kleidung manchmal mehr nach äußeren modischen Gesichtspunkten oder nach dem, was ihnen am besten steht, als nach innerem Gefühl. Oft ist dabei aber nur die äußere Kleidung modisch gefärbt, während direkt auf der Haut getragene Kleidungsstücke doch die eigentliche Farbe zeigen. Dann kann die Wahl eines Edelsteins Klarheit bringen, denn der entspricht farblich eher dem inneren Gefühl. Wir haben zu diesem Zweck eine Steinsammlung in Form eines Farbkreises angelegt. Männer nennen ihre Farbvorliebe manchmal als Autofarbe, wenn man praktische Gesichtspunkte wie Schmutzempfindlichkeit etc. abstrahiert.
- *Unentschlossen:* Nachdem zwei oder drei Farben gewählt wurden, es aber unentschieden ist, welche eigentlich bevorzugt wird, lässt man die Farben direkt vergleichen. Die dann bevorzugte notieren wir als erste. Oft bringt aber erst eine später wiederholte Farbwahl Klarheit.
- *Kunstmaler etc:* Wer beruflich mit Farben zu tun hat oder hobbymäßig malt, hat oft Schwierigkeiten mit der Farbvorliebe. Manchmal klärt sich die Frage durch häufigere Wiederholung des Farbtests, aber oft bleibt die Farbvorliebe unklar.
- *Farbenblindheit:* Auch Farbenblinde wählen oft eine Farbe aus. Ihre homöopathische Gültigkeit scheint unklar.

Klinische Zuverlässigkeit der Farbvorliebe als homöopathisches Symptom

Im Juli 2003 machten wir eine retrospektive Studie mit 450 Kindern bis 13 Jahren, die in den letzten 6 Jahren in unserer Praxis mit einem Einzelmittel erfolgreich behandelt wurden. Von diesen 450 Kindern wurden 160 mit der üblichen homöopathischen Methode und ohne Hinzuziehung der Farbvorliebe geheilt oder gebessert. Die übrigen 290 Kinder waren alt genug und gewillt, eine Farbe auszuwählen, die sie gerne mochten.

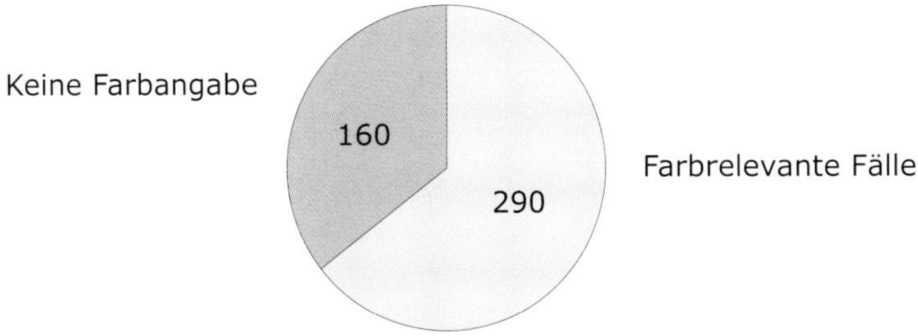

Gesamtübersicht aller Fälle
n = 450

Aus dieser Gesamtzahl von 290 farbrelevanten Fällen wurden 160 mit Hilfe der Farbvorliebe gelöst. Mit anderen Worten wurden ungefähr 55% dieser 290 Kinder mit einem Mittel geheilt oder gebessert, welches mit Beteiligung der Farbvorliebe ausgewählt wurde, d. h. eine von zwei gewählten Farben stimmte mit der bekannten Farbvorliebe des Heilmittels überein. In ungefähr 30% von 290 farbrelevanten Fällen wäre das gegebene Mittel ohne das Farbsymptom nicht gefunden worden. In diesen Fällen öffnete also die Farbvorliebe das Fenster zum Heilmittel. Und in ungefähr 25% war die Farbvorliebe ein Begleitsymptom, das die auf übliche Weise getroffene Mittelwahl stützte. In diesen Fällen hätte man also das Mittel auch auf gängigem Wege finden können, wenn auch mit einem größeren Unsicherheitsfaktor. In den restlichen 45% stimmte die Farbvorliebe des einzelnen Kindes mit der bisher bekannten Farbe des Mittels nicht überein. Wir glauben nicht, dass diese Zahlen bedeuten, dass man die Erfolgsrate durch Hinzuziehung der Farbvorliebe um 30% steigern könnte. Das wäre enorm, doch wir meinen, dass wir auch auf anderen Wegen zu guten Mitteln für diese Kinder gefunden hätten, wenn auch vielleicht nicht zu so guten.

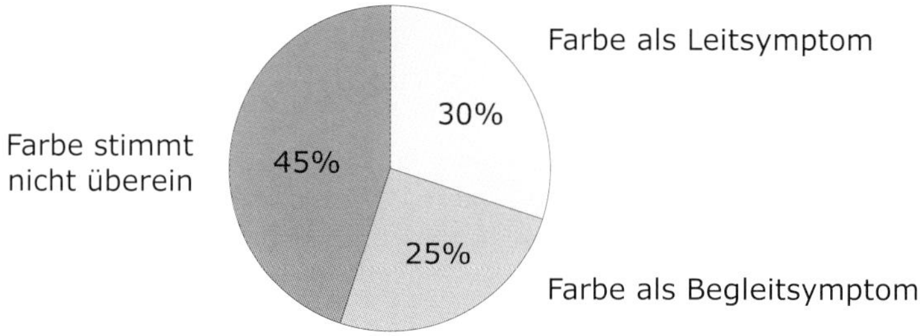

Farbrelevante Fälle
n = 290

Um die genannten Zahlen zu widerlegen oder zu bestätigen, wäre eine unabhängige Überprüfung durch erfahrene Homöopathen nötig. Da wir die bekannten Farbvorlieben nutzten, waren wir natürlich geneigt, sie als gegeben anzunehmen und nach ihnen zu verschreiben, wenn auch mit gutem Erfolg. Es wäre interessant, die nachträglich erhobenen Farbvorlieben von geheilten Patienten anderer Ärzte zu erhalten. Wir würden eine solche Kooperation sehr begrüßen.

Ändert sich die Farbvorliebe?

Ja, das gibt es oft. Wir haben es besonders bei Kindern beobachtet. Ihre Farbwahl ist meist leicht und natürlich. Man mag den Farbtest öfter wiederholen, doch sie bleiben manchmal jahrelang bei ihrer Farbe, bis sie sich plötzlich ändert. Sie treten nun offenbar in eine andere Entwicklungsphase ein. Wir sehen dies auch als Hinweis auf andere Mittelgruppen.

Calendula: Wir wollen ein Beispiel nehmen. Ein dreijähriges Mädchen kam mit multiplen linsengroßen, verhärteten, rot entzündeten Hautknoten in beiden Leisten, Ellbeugen und Kniekehlen. Diese Knoten bestanden seit 9 Monaten, und die Entzündung nahm zu. 6 Monate vor dieser Erkrankung litt sie an Mollusken in den Kniekehlen, die nach mehreren vergeblichen Therapieversuchen in Vollnarkose operiert wurden. Die Vollnarkose war nötig, weil sie sich dermaßen vehement wehrte, dass selbst 3 ausgewachsene Männer nicht ausreichten, um sie stillzuhalten. Sie hat eine ausgeprägte Abneigung gegen Berührung von Männern und ganz besonders von ihrem Vater, der merkwürdigerweise eine über den ganzen Körper verteilte Vitiligo hat. Er durfte sie morgens nicht einmal ansehen. Sie wirkte verfeinert, charmant, eigenwillig und wollte nicht, dass man ihr irgendwie in die Quere kam. Sie liebte Barbiepuppen und wollte eine Prinzessin sein. Sie fürchtete sich sehr vor plötzlichen durchdringenden Schreien. Sie hatte eine ausgeprägte Abneigung vor Eiern. Sie wählte als Farbvorliebe 11 B, ein helles Pink. Sie bekam Calendula 1000 aufgrund der Asteraceae-Themen ihres Verhaltens (eigenwillige Abwehrhaltung etc., siehe Scholtens Beschreibung der Korbblütler) und ihrer Farbvorliebe, die auf diese spezielle Variante der Asteraceae hinwies. Zugegeben war die Verschreibung nur ein Versuch, über die nur als Wundmittel bekannte Calendula mehr zu erfahren, denn die dürftigen Prüfungssymptome lieferten keine ausreichende Begründung für die Verordnung. Aber die Ringelblume wirkte ausgezeichnet. Nach 3 Tagen begannen die Knoten abzublassen und kleiner zu werden. Dann hatte sie eine Nacht hohes Fieber, ohne sich krank zu fühlen. Darauf änderte sich ihr Verhalten gegen den Vater. Sie ging auf ihn zu und freute sich, wenn er sie in den Arm nahm. Er war so erstaunt, dass er meinte, man hätte sie irgendwie unter Drogen gesetzt. Auch begann sie plötzlich Eier zu essen und hatte weniger Angst vor plötzlichen lauten Schreien.

Sie blieb 7 Monate lang bei der gleichen Farbvorliebe und wechselte dann zu 17 C, einem Blautürkis oder Cyan. Der Farbwechsel fiel in eine Zeit, in der der Vater die Familie verließ und auszog. Damals entwickelte sie ein Ekzem am Brustkorb. Weil sich der Vater von der Familie zurückzog und sie alleine ließ[1] und diese Situation vermutlich das Ekzem auslöste, bekam sie Nat-sil 1000. Auch die neue Farbvorliebe wies als Begleitsymptom auf ein Mittel aus der Natriumgruppe hin. Innerhalb von 2 Wochen ging das Ekzem weg, und seit nunmehr einem halben Jahr geht es ihr völlig gut.

Bei manchen Erwachsenen ändert sich die Farbvorliebe häufig, bei anderen bleibt sie sehr lange konstant oder hält für ein ganzes Leben. Es mag sein, dass solche Menschen ihren endgültigen Stil gefunden haben, es mag aber auch sein, dass ihre Entwicklung stehenblieb, weil sie der Macht der Gewohnheit verfielen und ihre jugendliche Kraft dahinging. Auch die zu häufige Wiederholung des Farbtests scheint bei manchen eine oberflächliche Änderung der Farbvorliebe auszulösen. Dann wird das Resultat immer zweifelhafter. Nach unserem Gefühl ist deren Farbe oft die zuallererst ausgesuchte, oder man könnte grün vermuten (siehe Farbkonzepte). Wer jedoch rot

---

[1] Siehe "Homöopathie und die Elemente" von Jan Scholten, unter Natrum silicatum.

oder blau mag, bleibt meist lange bei seiner Farbe, selbst wenn man häufig danach fragt.

Abneigung gegen eine Farbe

Manche Menschen haben eine eindeutige Abneigung gegen eine Farbe, die sich genauso exakt bestimmen läßt wie die Farbvorliebe. Einige unserer Fälle bestätigen, dass man hier die gleichen Mittel berücksichtigen kann, die für die Vorliebe gelten. Immerhin ist sie nur der andere Pol derselben Achse. Aber wir haben nicht systematisch nach Abneigungen gefragt und damit weniger Erfahrung mit dieser Information. Weitere Fälle weisen darauf hin, dass auch ein intermittierender Wechsel von Zuneigung und Abneigung gegen eine bestimmte Farbe auf die Mittel dieser Farbe hinweist. Ähnliches mag für die Wahl einer Komplementärfarbe gelten, also einer Farbe, die im Farbkreis in Opposition steht. Das ist im Moment noch reine Spekulation. Wenn jemand diesbezüglich eigene Erfahrungen hat, würde es uns sehr interessieren.

Wie entdeckt man die Farbvorliebe eines Mittels?

Im Laufe von 15 Jahren wurden bei schätzungsweise 20 000 Patienten die Farbvorlieben bestimmt. Aus dieser Gesamtzahl trugen etwa 3000 Patienten zur Entdeckung der Farbzuordnung bei.

Cichorium: Nehmen wir als Beispiel ein recht unbekanntes Mittel, dessen Farbvorliebe bislang noch unbekannt war: Cichorium intybus, die Wegwarte. Unsere zuvor genannte Übersicht über 450 Kinderfälle zeigte, dass wir 227 verschiedene Einzelmittel verwendet hatten. Das am häufigsten gegebene Mittel war Belladonna mit 10 erfolgreichen Fällen, doch Cichorium und Cina folgten dicht mit je 9 Fällen. Neun Kinder, die mit demselben Mittel geheilt wurden, sind eine aussichtsreiche Zahl, um die Farbe des Mittels herauszufinden. Wir verglichen nun ihre Farbvorlieben, die wir ähnlich wie Nahrungsmodalitäten systematisch bei jeder Anamnese erheben. 6 von diesen 9 "Cichorium-Kindern" hatten ihre Farben angeben können, die restlichen 3 waren noch zu klein dafür. Das Kind, welches am besten auf Cichorium angesprochen hatte, hatte mehrfach ein ganz zartes Zitronengelb gewählt, 1 A in unserem neuen Buch. Der zweitbeste Fall hatte genau die gleiche Farbe gewählt, und eines von 5 weiteren gut auf Cichorium reagierenden Kindern wählte ein kräftigeres Zitronengelb 1 C. Ein weiterer recht guter Fall wählte dunkelblau, und ein nur mäßig ansprechendes Kind suchte ein dunkles Violett aus, beides ungefähr komplementäre Farben zu gelb (siehe Abneigung gegen eine Farbe). Also schälte sich gelb als Farbvorliebe von Cichorium heraus, und um genauer zu sein ein helles zartes Zitronengelb 1 A oder 1 C.

Das Leitsymptom zur Verschreibung des Mittels war Scholtens Information der unerwünschten Schwangerschaft in Kombination mit weiteren Charakteristika der botanischen Familie der Asteraceae oder Compositae. Dieses Symptom wurde in 6 von 9 Fällen bestätigt. Die Mütter hatten während der Schwangerschaft eine Abtreibung des Kindes erwogen. Vier dieser Kinder schrieen laut und mit durchdringend unangenehmer Stimme. Sie forderten Aufmerksamkeit und zwangen der Umgebung oft lärmend ihren Willen auf. Ferner neigten sie alle häufig zu sehr hohem Fieber. 7 der 9 Fälle waren gute Fälle, die nicht nur oberflächlich angesprochen hatten. Also fügten wir Cich im zweiten Grad in die Farbliste unter 1 A ein (dieser Repertoriumsgrad bedeutet, dass die Farbe durch mindestens 2 gute Fälle bestätigt wurde). Bei Bestätigung der Farbe durch weitere Fälle kommt das Mittel in den dritten Grad.

Die Gefahr der Überschätzung der Farbvorliebe

Bei den genannten Cichorium-Fällen gab es natürlich keine Voreingenommenheit zugunsten der Farbvorliebe als Hilfe zur Mittelwahl, weil die Farbe des Mittels noch gar nicht bekannt war und die Verschreibung nach üblichen Gesichtspunkten erfolgte. Bei den Belladonna-Fällen war jedoch eine gewisse "Farblastigkeit" zugunsten der bekannten Farbvorliebe, eines warmen Butterblumengelb, nicht zu übersehen. Ein homöopathischer Kollege, der gerade seine ersten Sporen bei uns verdiente, verschrieb das Mittel oft und gern, weil er die Leichtigkeit des Farbsymptoms schätzen gelernt hatte. Das Resultat waren 4 ordentliche Fälle mittlerer Qualität, die z.B. ein paar bekannte Symptome verifizierten, eine isolierte geistige Verbesserung herbeiführten oder eine rezidivierende Otitis heilten, ohne jedoch tiefere Veränderungen zu hinterlassen. Die Verschreibung nach Schlüsselsymptomen als Abkürzung des homöopathischen Verfahrens ist einer von vielen möglichen homöopathischen Wegen, doch hängt der Erfolg sehr von der Qualität der verwendeten keynotes ab und setzt voraus, dass die Essenz des Falles richtig verstanden wurde. Wer sich von der Farbvorliebe verführen lässt und sich zu sehr auf sie verlässt, wird oft nur oberflächliche Wirkungen sehen.

Studium eines Mittels durch geheilte Fälle

Die retrospektive Analyse eines wirklich guten Falles macht uns das eingesetzte Mittel oft erst so richtig plastisch. Besonders ergiebig ist die Meta-Analyse mehrerer Fälle des gleichen Mittels. Warum sollten wir uns ausschließlich auf die Arzneimittelprüfungen verlassen? Viele neue Charakteristika homöopathischer Mittel lassen sich auch durch die klinische Methode finden, vorausgesetzt wir studieren nur die wirklich guten Fälle. Die gesamten Farbzuordnungen wurden so gefunden. Sie stammen also nicht aus Prüfungen, doch sie ergänzen den Reichtum der Prüfungssymptome. H.V. Müller entdeckte hunderte von Farbzuordnungen durch die klinische Methode. Wir konnten viele durch schöne Heilerfolge verifizieren. Die komplette Liste einschließlich aller Suchmittel, die bislang nur durch einen schönen Fall bestätigt sind, umfaßt inzwischen ungefähr 700 Mittel. Wir haben eigene Erfahrungen mit ca. 550 von ihnen, und der Rest gibt ausschließlich die Erfahrungen H.V. Müllers weiter.

Farbvorliebe und Handschrift

Die Farbvorliebe ist ein subtiles Symptom und kann sich einem Zugriff oft geschickt entziehen. Ihre Feststellung ist mit mehreren Unsicherheitsfaktoren belastet (siehe Schwierigkeiten). So begann Müller nach einem ebenso umfassenden, aber solideren Symptom zu suchen, das wie die Farbvorliebe tiefere Schichten der Persönlichkeit wiedergibt. Dabei kam er auf die Handschrift. Er begann sich von jedem Patienten eine standardisierte Schriftprobe auf einem unlinierten DIN A 4 Blatt geben zu lassen und fand ähnliche Schriftstrukturen bei Personen, die mit demselben Heilmittel geheilt wurden[2]. Seit Anfang der 90er Jahre begann er die Farbvorliebe mit der Handschrift zu kombinieren, um bei der üblichen Repertorisation eines Falles durch Hinzuziehung dieser Verbindung zweier persönlichkeitsrelevanter Symptome größere Genauigkeit in der Verschreibung zu erzielen. In späteren Jahren definierte Müller die Farbvorliebe eines Mittels nur, wenn er mindestens zwei oder drei gute Fälle eines Mittels hatte, die nicht nur die Farbvorliebe teilten, sondern auch ähnliche Schriftzüge aufwiesen. Man muss allerdings sehen, dass damit die Definition der

---

[2] Man kann vermuten, dass auf diese Weise noch weitere mittelspezifische Charakteristika gefunden werden können, wie z.B. Beziehungen zu Blutgruppen, mittelspezifische Ähnlichkeiten des Fingerabdrucks, der DNA-Sequenzen, Handlinien, Irismuster etc.

Farbvorliebe nicht nur präzisiert, sondern auch ziemlich eingeengt wird.

Wir tauschten in brieflicher Korrespondenz viele kopierte Patientenhandschriften aus, die nach folgendem Muster abgefasst waren: In der Schriftprobe schildert der Patient seine Hauptbeschwerden oder schreibt einen standardisierten Text ab. Auf der Rückseite des unlinierten DIN A 4 Blattes notieren wir die medizinische Diagnose, die Farbvorlieben und die homöopathische Begründung des erfolgreichen Mittels (charakteristische Rubriken, Materia Medica Symptome, botanische Konzepte, Serien und Stadien, Miasmen etc). An dieser Stelle mehr darüber zu sagen, würde den gegebenen Rahmen unseres Themas sprengen. Wir beabsichtigen darüber ein weiteres Buch zu schreiben.

Kann ein Mittel mehrere Farbvorlieben haben?

H.V. Müller war überzeugt, dass jedes Mittel nur einer einzigen Farbe zugeordnet werden sollte. Daher sind die meisten Mittel in der Liste nur unter einer einzigen Farbe zu finden. Es gibt jedoch gute Gründe, dies anders zu sehen:

Bambusa arundinacea: Wir haben 11 Frauen erfolgreich mit Bambus behandelt. Die Verschreibungen erfolgten aufgrund einer ausgezeichneten Arzneimittelprüfung, die nicht nur zuverlässige Prüfungssymptome angibt, sondern auch klinische Fälle beschreibt, die die Prüfungssymptome verifizieren. Durch unsere 11 Patientinnen fanden wir nicht nur die Farbvorliebe von Bambus, ein reines Lapislazuliblau 15-16 C, sondern sie wiesen auch Ähnlichkeiten in der Handschrift auf und ließen sich in zwei gut abgrenzbare Schrifttypen unterteilen. Sechs Frauen wählten reines Blau als erste Farbe. Drei weitere wählten blau als Zweitfarbe, eine von ihnen als dunkelblau 15 D. Es gab eine weitere auffallende Häufung der Farbe schwarz. Drei wählten schwarz als erste Farbe, und diese drei waren es auch, die blau als Zweitfarbe wählten. Weitere genannte Farben waren wahllos verteilt bis auf eine fragliche dritte Häufung von grün 20 C, nur zweimal genannt. Warum sollte man also nur blau als einzige Farbvorliebe für Bambus angeben? Schwarz gehört als Zweitfarbe dazu, wenn auch weniger ausgeprägt als blau.

Die beiden Farbvorlieben blau und schwarz treffen auch für Titan zu, doch diese Patienten haben eine andere Handschrift. Bei Manganum phosphoricum sahen wir gute Fälle sowohl mit reinem Rot als auch mit dunklem Magenta als Farbvorliebe. Nur weitere Beobachtungen werden zeigen können, wie ausgeprägt die angegebenen Farbzuordnungen wirklich sind. Vielleicht gibt es bei einzelnen Mitteln verschiedene Farbspitzen, oder eine Kombination zweier Farbvorlieben charakterisiert das Mittel. Müller analysierte seine Fälle in der gleichen Weise, wie wir es hier am Beispiel von Bambus gezeigt haben, doch er gab immer nur eine Farbvorliebe an, vielleicht um weitere Komplikationen zu vermeiden.

Wie wenden wir die Farbvorliebe praktisch an?

- *Als normales Allgemeinsymptom:* Meistens verwenden wir die Farbvorliebe wie jedes andere Allgemein- oder Gemütssymptom, mit der nötigen Reserve und der Bereitschaft, sie jederzeit zurückzustellen, wenn bessere Symptome in eine andere Richtung weisen. Wir berücksichtigen dabei auch, mit welcher Gewissheit der Patient die Farbe nannte.
- *In Kombination mit der Handschrift:* Man kann bei der Mittelsuche die Handschriften aller Mittel vergleichen, die durch die Farbvorliebe vorgeschlagen werden (natürlich braucht man dazu eine Handschriftensammlung). Wenn man darunter eine ähnliche Schrift entdeckt und dieses Mittel mit seinen allgemeinen Charakteristika der Idee des vorliegenden Falles entspricht, so hat man hohe Gewissheit für eine gute Verschreibung.
- *Zur Differenzierung ähnlicher Mittel:* Nehmen wir an, wir sollen einen Fall lösen, bei dem die Differenzierung zwischen Belladonna und Stramonium schwerfällt. Wenn die Farbvorliebe rot ist, geben wir Stramonium, wenn sie gelb ist Belladonna.
- *Zur Findung "kleiner Arzneimittel":* Wer vorwiegend Polychreste verschreibt, wird durch die Farbvorliebe oft auf kleine Mittel hingewiesen werden, die selten verordnet werden. Diese Mittel sind aber nur deshalb klein, weil sie im Repertorium selten auftauchen, oder anders gesagt weil die Polychreste im Repertorium überrepräsentiert sind.
- *In der Computerrepertorisation:* Man kann die Farben als Rubriken ins Computerrepertorium nachtragen, doch wenn man als Analysestrategie die kleinen Mittel aufwertet, werden viele Mittel der Farbrubrik überbewertet und stehen im

Ergebnis an erster Stelle, auch wenn sonst überhaupt nichts für sie spricht. Man lasse sich dadurch nicht irreführen.

- *Als Rettungsanker:* Unter erschwerten Umständen wie z.B. bei einer Anamnese ohne Kenntnis der Sprache des Patienten kann die Farbvorliebe manchmal rettend sein. In Indien konnten wir diese Erfahrung machen, und die Validität des Farbsymptoms war überraschend hoch. Mehrere Dutzend dieser Fälle wurden in Homeopathic LINKS 1/01 publiziert.

Farbkonzepte

Hierin erblicken wir den Schlüssel zu einem zukünftigen natürlichen System der Stimmungen und Funktionen der Lebenskraft und damit auch zu einer natürlichen Gliederung der homöopathischen Materia Medica. Wir unterscheiden 4 Hauptfarben: gelb, rot, blau, grün; 3 Zwischenfarben: orange, violett, türkis; 2 Nebenfarben: braun, olive; sowie schwarz und weiss, und deren Zwischenstufe grau. Somit ergeben sich bis zu 12 Gruppen, die wir als Farbkonzepte definieren können.

Über die Einteilung und Bedeutung der Farben wurde seit alten Zeiten viel gemutmaßt und wenig Übereinstimmendes behauptet. Kulturelle Unterschiede spielen hier bestimmt auch mit. Es gibt wenige wissenschaftliche Untersuchungen darüber, und nur die Zuordnungen von rot und blau scheinen relativ sicher. Die folgenden Themen geben teilweise H.V. Müllers Erfahrungen und zum Teil unsere eigenen Beobachtungen wieder. Besonders die Zwischenfarben sind uns noch nicht richtig klar, so dass wir sie ausgelassen haben. Aber auch die genannten Farbkonzepte betrachten wir nur als Arbeitshypothese.

Rot Aktiv Vorwärtsdenken, progressiv Revolution Opportunismus Leidenschaftliche Liebe Feuer, Hitze	**Blau** Empfänglich Rückblick, Geschichte Reaktion Klassisch, zuverlässig, konservativ Langweilig Wasser, kühlend
Grün Veränderlich Vielfalt Ambivalent Fernreisen Assimilation, Wachstum	**Gelb** Vorstellungskraft Inspiriert, high Hellsichtig Unstet, flüchtig Ohne festen Boden
Schwarz Nein Unabhängig Folgt eigenem Gesetz Hart Dunkle Macht	**Weiß** Rein wie Schnee Löst sich von Leidenschaft Löscht Unterschiede aus Verhärtet Radikal

Schlusswort

Abschließend wollen wir noch einige persönliche Gedanken anfügen. Welche Motive und Umstände führten zu diesem Buch? Als Kinder der Sechzigerjahre begegneten wir uns in der Aufbruchstimmung der Hippiezeit, und die Ideen, die Musik und die Kunst dieser Epoche waren überall lebendig. Wir machten uns wenig Gedanken, dass uns das Schicksal in der Zukunft als homöopathische Gemeinschaftspraxis zusammenfügen würde und sich unsere Erfahrungen in diesem Buch kristallisieren sollten. Die eigentliche Sehnsucht galt der Freiheit durch Bewusstseinserweiterung und der religiösen Erfahrung. Damals trafen wir einen Menschen, der ein eigenständiger Denker und Schriftsteller war und in seiner Person die höchsten spirituellen Erfahrungen verwirklicht hatte, die er voller Freude und Bescheidenheit mitzuteilen wusste. Sein Name war Swami Narayanananda, und er maß der Existenz einer Lebenskraft, die er Kundalini Shakti nannte, große Bedeutung bei. Als dynamischer Aspekt des ruhenden Bewusstseins ist sie der Ursprung des Geistes und bewahrt unsere Erfahrungen in kausaler Form auf, die damit als Gedächtnis zur Verfügung stehen. Die Geistesfunktionen hängen völlig von dieser Lebenskraft ab. Sie ist gleichzeitig die zentrale Kraft des Körpers, sein eigentliches Leben, und alle vitalen Funktionen hängen von ihr ab. Ohne diese Lebenskraft haben Körper und Geist keine eigenständige Existenz[3].

Als wir wenige Jahre später sahen, wie eng Hahnemanns Beschreibungen der Lebenskraft mit den Erkenntnissen dieses Heiligen übereinstimmten, war es nur natürlich, dass wir uns während des Medizinstudiums Mitte der Siebzigerjahre der Homöopathie zuwandten, bevor wir 1983 in Kandern unsere Gemeinschaftspraxis gründeten.

Hahnemanns Vorstellung von Krankheit als primär dynamische "Verstimmung" der Lebenskraft, die sich sekundär durch geistige und körperliche Symptome kundgibt, hat bis in unsere Zeit für zahlreiche Kontroversen gesorgt. Das dürfte zum großen Teil an der Unfähigkeit vieler Menschen liegen, zum Verständnis der Lebenskraft ihr Vorstellungsvermögen von mechanischen Ideen freizumachen. Die Lebenskraft hat kein Gewicht und keine Größe, denn sie ist selbst die

3 Weitere Details finden sich in dem Buch "Die Urkraft im Menschen oder die Kundalini Shakti" von Swami Narayanananda.

Ursache von Zeit und Raum und entzieht sich ihnen damit. Dennoch kann man sie bis zu einem gewissen Grad verstehen, denn ein klarer Geist und ein reines Herz spiegeln sie als eigenen Ursprung, als eigenes Selbst, wieder.

Die Idee der Farbvorliebe als einfaches und doch tiefes Symptom der persönlichen Neigung sprach uns sofort an. Ohne großen Aufwand gibt sie zwanglos die innere Verfassung des Patienten wieder und schlägt uns direkt einige dazu passende Mittel vor. Die Farbvorliebe ist allgemeiner als ein Lokalsymptom und allgemeiner als eine spezifische Verkennung (basic delusion) der eigenen Lage; Sankarans neueste homöopathische Forschungen über "sensations" und "energy patterns", Grundmuster der Empfindung, die als Familienthemen der Botanik homöopathisch interpretierbar werden, weisen in eine ähnliche Richtung. Die Farbvorliebe ist eine einfache Neigung des Geistes und gibt direkt die individuelle Schwingung oder Stimmung der Lebenskraft wieder. Andere würden sagen, dass sie die individuelle Aura anzeigt. Diese Schwingung färbt gewissermaßen den Geist und erzeugt beim Anblick der entsprechenden Farben eine freudige Wiedererkennung, oder auch eine instinktive Ablehnung, falls eine Dissonanz wahrgenommen wird. Die Farbvorliebe ist natürlich keine Krankheit. Wie aber eine bestimmte Pflanze sich eine passende Bodenbeschaffenheit aussucht, so können auch bestimmte Krankheiten mit einer zugehörigen Disposition zusammenhängen.

Lieber Leser! Nun sind wir am Ende unserer Geschichte angelangt, und sie hätte ihren Sinn erfüllt, wenn das Buch als Werkzeug angewendet wird und eigene Erfahrungen mit der Methode entstehen. Mögen sie dazu führen, den Patienten mit der Homöopathie noch besser helfen zu können!

Burgberg, im August 2003

Ulrich Welte & Herbert Sigwart

Transformation of H.V. Müller's Color Codes from "Taschenlexikon der Farben"

(Umwandlungstabelle für die früheren Farbcodes)

	A	B	C	D	E
1	1-2 A 2-3	1-2 A 4-5	1-2 A 6-8	1-2 BCD 8	1-2 EF 8
2	3 A 2-3	3 A 4-5	3 A 6-8	3 BC 8	3 DEF 8
3	4 A 2-3	4 A 4-6	4 A 7-8	4 BC 8	4 DEF 8
4	5-6 A 2-3	5-6 A 4-6	5-6 A 7-8	5-6 BCD 8	5-6 EF 8
5	7 A 2-3	7 A 4-6	7 A 7-8	7 BCD 8	7 EF 8
6	8 A 2-3	8 A 4-6	8 A 7-8	8 BCD 8	8 EF 8
7	9 A 2-3	9 A 4-6	9 AB 7-8	9 CD 8	9 EF 8
8	10 A 2-3	10 A 4-6	10 AB 7-8	10 CD 8	10 EF 8
9	11 A 2-3	11 A 4-6	11 AB 7-8	11 CD 8	11 EF 8
10	12 A 2-3	12 A 4-7	12 AB 8	12 CD 8	12 EF 8
11	13-14 A 2-4	13-14 A 5-7	13-14 AB 8	13-14 CD 8	13-14 EF 8
12	15 A 2-3	15 A 4-6	15 AB 7-8	15 CD 8	15 EF 8
13	16-17 A 2-3	16-17 A 4-6	16-17 AB 7-8	16-17 CD 8	16-17 EF 8
14	18 A 2-3	18 A 4-7	18 AB 8	18 CD 8	18 EF 8
15	19-20 A 2-3	19-20 A 4-6	19-20 AB 7-8	19-20 CD 8	19-20 EF 8
16	21-22 A 2-3	21-22 A 4-6	21-22 AB 7-8	21-22 CD 8	21-22 EF 8
17	23 A 2-3	23 A 4-6	23 AB 7-8	23 CD 8	23 EF 8
18	24 A 2-3	24 A 4-6	24 AB 7-8	24 CD 8	24 EF 8
19	25 A 2-3	25 A 4-6	25 A 7-8	25 BCD 8	25 EF 8
20	26 A 2-3	26 A 4-6	26 AB 7-8	26 CD 8	26 EF 8
21	26-27 A 2-3	26-27 A 4-6	26-27 AB 7-8	26-27 CD 8	26-27 EF 8
22	27 A 2-3	27 A 4-7	27 AB 8	27 CD 8	27 EF 8
23	28-29 A 2-3	28-29 A 4-6	28-29 A 7-8	28-29 BCD 8	28-29 EF 8
24	30 A 2-4	30 A 5-6	30 A 7-8	30 BCD 8	30 EF 8

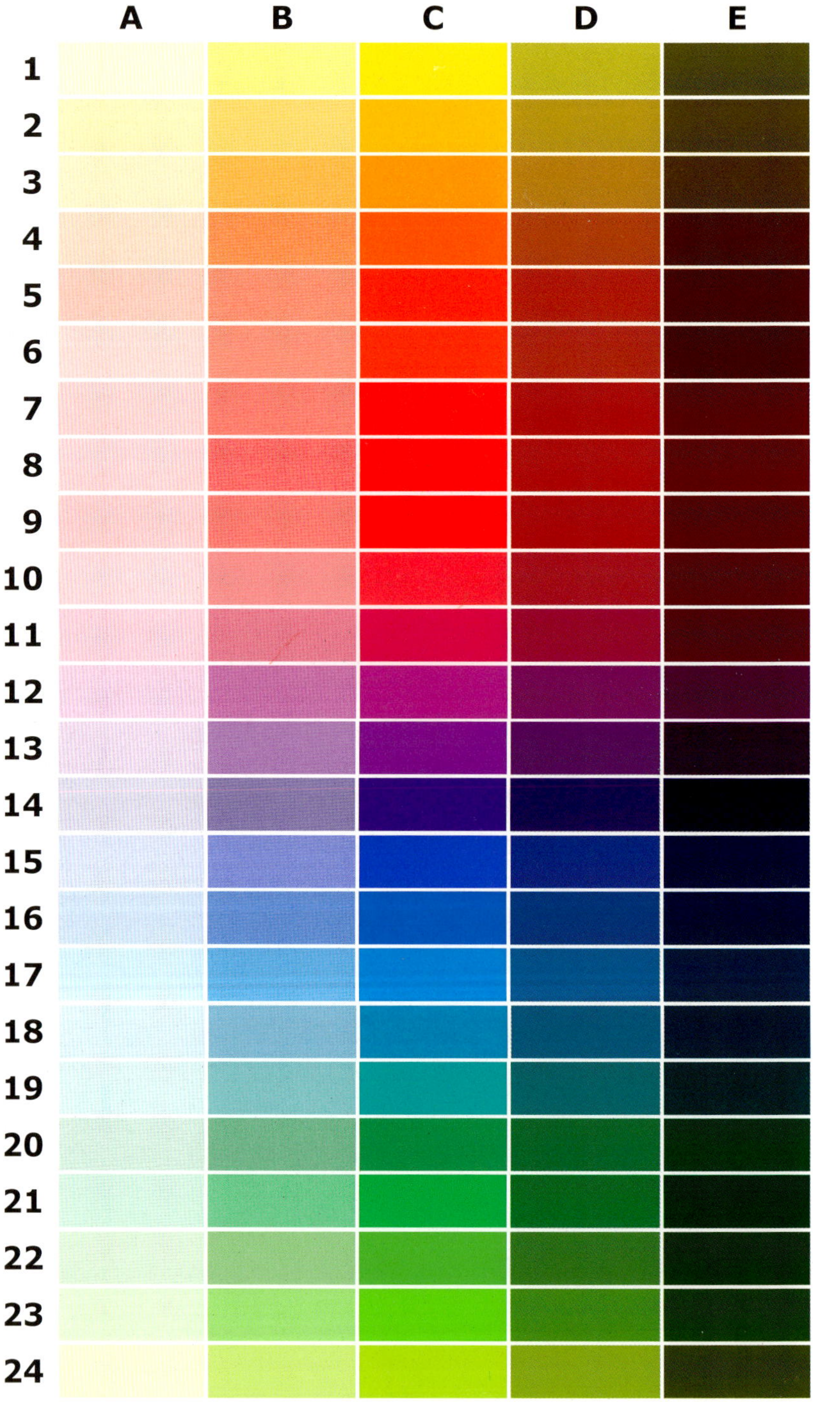
A
B
C
D
E
1
2
3
4
5
6
7
8
9
10
11
12
13
14
15
16
17
18
19
20
21
22
23
24

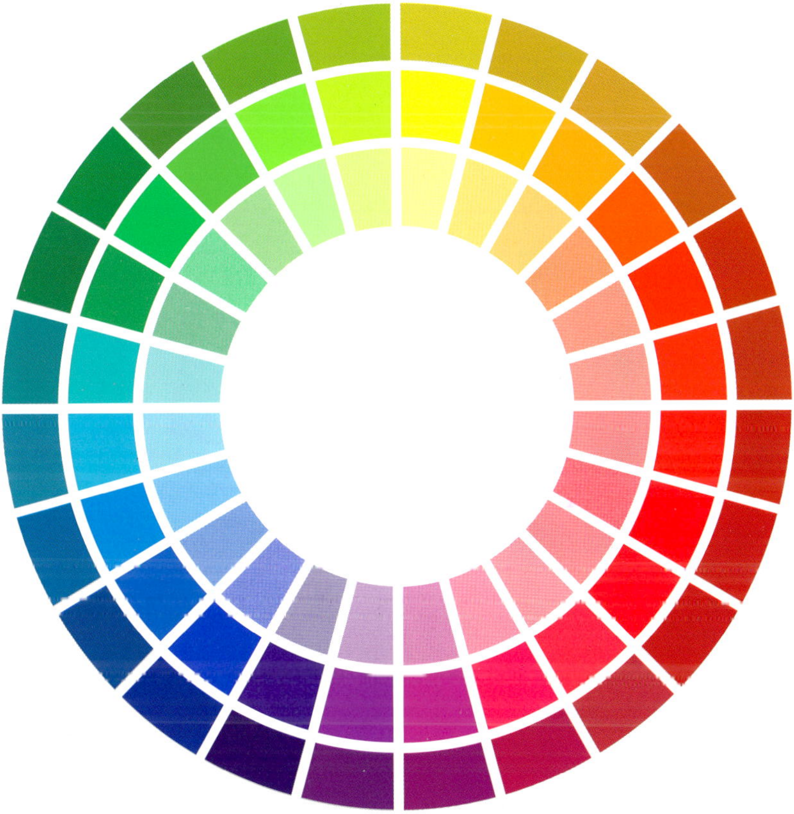

From the Foreword by Jan Scholten

The color preference is a significant and effective symptom. It's effective in the sense that it can give the indication or confirmation of a diagnosis in many cases. The color preference is a peculiar symptom expressing the in[illegible]e patient, which is the state of the remedy. And it's a [illegible]nptom.

The table designed b[illegible] best usable I've seen till now. All colors are cl[illegible]tandardised, so it can be used in the future with[illegible]

Aus dem Vorwort von Jan Scholten

Die Farbvorliebe ist ein signifikantes und effektives Symptom. Effektiv in dem Sinne, daß sie in vielen Fällen eine Arzneimitteldiagnose anzeigen oder bestätigen kann. Die Farbvorliebe ist ein charakteristisches Symptom, das den inneren Zustand des Patienten und damit auch die Natur des Arzneimittels ausdrückt. Außerdem ist sie als Symptom sehr spezifisch.

Die Farbtabelle von Ulrich Welte ist die praktischste, die ich bisher gesehen habe. Alle Farben sind klar und genau standardisiert. Damit wird man sich in Zukunft unzweideutig auf sie beziehen können.